PREGNANCY GUIDE FOR MEN

Ideal Guide to become a fantastic Dad and support your partner during Pregnancy to create a strong and happy Family by eradicating false fear and anxiety

Diego Moore

Table of Contents

All rights reserved

Copyright ©2023 by Diego Moore. All rights reserved.

PREGNANCY GUIDE FOR MEN

Bonus

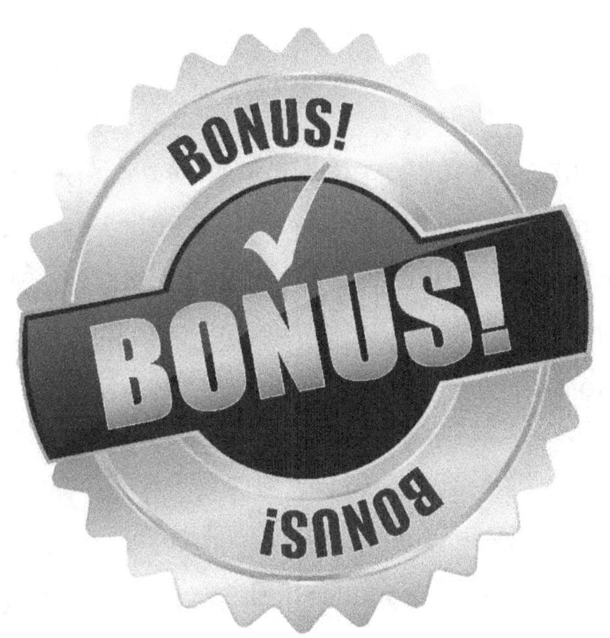

Hi future Dad!

Scan the QR Code and enjoy your free bonus!

GET YOUR FREE GIFT

Introduction

Becoming a father is one of life's most transformative and awe-inspiring experiences. It's a journey that begins with anticipation, is marked by countless precious moments, and continues to unfold with each passing day. The moment you learn you are going to be a father, the world seems to shift, offering you a new perspective on life, love, and responsibility. This guide is crafted especially for you, the expectant father, as you step into this incredible adventure called fatherhood.

Acknowledgments

Before we delve into the heart of this guide, it's important to express gratitude to those who have contributed to its creation. The wisdom and experiences shared by countless fathers, mothers, and parenting experts have enriched the content you're about to explore. We acknowledge the invaluable insights and support provided by these individuals, whose collective knowledge has made this guide possible.

About This Book

Pregnancy Guide for Men is more than just a book—it is a trusted resource, a source of inspiration, and a companion on your journey into fatherhood. Whether you are eagerly awaiting the arrival of your child or have already cradled your newborn in your arms, this guide is designed to offer valuable insights, practical advice, and heartfelt encouragement.

This book is divided into chapters that mirror the various stages of fatherhood, from the discovery of pregnancy to the challenges and joys of parenting through the years. Each chapter delves into specific aspects of the father's role, offering guidance on how to navigate the complexities of parenthood with confidence and grace.

How to Use This Guide

This comprehensive guide is organized to help you navigate your journey into fatherhood effectively. Here's how to make the most of it:

1. **Sequential Reading:** You can read this guide sequentially, starting from the Introduction and moving through each chapter in order. This approach provides a structured and comprehensive understanding of the fatherhood journey, from pregnancy to the postpartum period and beyond.

2. **Topic-Specific Exploration:** If you have specific questions or are facing particular challenges related to fatherhood, feel free to jump to the chapters or sections that address those concerns. Each chapter is designed to stand alone, offering guidance on specific topics.

3. **Ongoing Reference:** Keep this guide on hand as an ongoing reference throughout your journey into fatherhood. As your child grows and new obstacles present themselves, you might find yourself going back to specific chapters..

4. **Share with Others:** Share this guide with fellow fathers, partners, or anyone who may benefit from its insights. Parenthood is a collective experience, and the wisdom contained within these pages can benefit both new and experienced fathers alike.

5. **Make Notes:** When you read, think about making notes or recording your ideas in a journal. Your personal experiences and insights are valuable additions to your journey as a father.

As you embark on this extraordinary journey of fatherhood, we invite you to immerse yourself in the pages ahead, celebrate the moments of pure love and connection, and find strength in the challenges you encounter. Welcome to the world of fatherhood; your journey has just begun.

Chapter 1:

Understanding the Journey Ahead

Welcome to Fatherhood

The moment you learn you are going to be a father, your world undergoes a profound transformation. It's a moment of joy, excitement, and perhaps a touch of nervousness, as you realize that your life is about to change in ways you could never have imagined. Greetings from parenting, an incredible adventure full of wonder, difficulties, and unending love.

It is crucial that you understand that you are not alone when you set out on your journey. Countless fathers before you have navigated the same uncharted waters, and they have emerged as pillars of strength, guidance, and support for their children. You are joining a timeless fraternity of fathers who have shaped the course of history, and your role is no less significant.

One of the most beautiful aspects of fatherhood is the opportunity it offers for growth and self-discovery. You will find that you possess reservoirs of patience, love, and resilience you never knew existed. Your child will be a source of inspiration, encouraging you to become the best version of yourself, day by day.

Fatherhood is not limited to biology; it's about the love, care, and unwavering commitment you offer to your child. It's about late-night feedings, diaper changes, soothing lullabies, and joyful laughter that fills your home. It's about being there for every milestone, from first steps to graduation day.

Embracing fatherhood means embracing the responsibility to nurture, protect, and guide your child. It means being a role model, demonstrating the values you want your child to embrace, and teaching them the essential lessons of life. Your deeds and words will serve as a compass for them, helping them to navigate the world's complexity.

As referring to being a parent, it is essential to keep in mind that nobody possesses every one of the correct solutions. Since every child is different, becoming a father is an ongoing learning process. You will make mistakes, but you will also learn and grow from them. Your love and dedication are the most significant gifts you can give to your child, and they will be felt deeply throughout their life.

Fatherhood is also about partnership. It's about sharing the joys and challenges with your partner, who is your greatest ally on this journey. Together, open communication, cooperation, and mutual support will fortify your bond and provide a solid basis for your family. Together, you will celebrate the triumphs and navigate the trials of parenthood.

Together, open communication, cooperation, and mutual support will fortify your bond and provide a solid basis for your family. Your child will carry your love and guidance with them, and your influence will ripple through generations. You are embarking on a journey that will shape not only your child's future but also the future of our world.

So, welcome to fatherhood—a journey that will test your limits, expand your heart, and bring immeasurable joy. It's a path of self-awareness, development, and unending love. As you hold your child in your arms for the first time, you will realize that you are now a part of something greater than yourself—a legacy of love and wisdom that will endure through the ages. Embrace this remarkable journey with an open heart, and may it bring you the profound fulfillment and happiness that only fatherhood can offer.

The Role of an Expectant Father

Becoming an expectant father is a transformative experience filled with excitement, anticipation, and a dash of anxiety. Your role during pregnancy is vital, and your involvement can significantly impact the well-being of both your partner and the unborn child. Take a closer look at the vital role that you play as a father-to-be.

6. **Emotional Support:** One of the most important roles you have during pregnancy is to provide emotional support. Your partner is going through a whirlwind of emotions – from joy and anticipation to occasional moments of doubt and fear. Be there to listen, offer encouragement, and validate her feelings. To help her feel less anxious and more loved, your assurance will be greatly appreciated.

7. **Active Participation:** Your active participation in the pregnancy journey is invaluable. Go with your significant other to prenatal visits. Attend classes on birthing and parenting together. By actively participating in these activities, you show that you are dedicated to being a hands-on parent in addition to learning invaluable lessons.

8. **Recognizing bodily Changes**: Learn about the changes your spouse is going through on a bodily level. Many changes occur throughout pregnancy, such as exhaustion, mood fluctuations, and morning sickness. Grasping these changes can enable you to empathize with her journey and respond with understanding, patience, and care.

9. **Creating a Nurturing and Supportive Environment:** Establish a loving and supportive atmosphere at home. Help with household chores, encourage relaxation, and ensure she has a comfortable space to rest. Physical and emotional well-being are closely intertwined, and by cultivating a positive environment, you make a significant contribution to her health and the baby's development.

10. **Encouraging Healthy Habits:** Promote a healthy lifestyle for both your partner and yourself. Promote a healthy diet, consistent exercise, and enough sleep. Steer clear of dangerous drugs like alcohol and smoke, and assist her in making these wise decision. Your proactive engagement in creating a conducive environment can result in a healthier pregnancy and a strong beginning for your child.

11. **Planning and Preparation:** Participate in planning for the baby's arrival. From choosing baby names to setting up the nursery, your involvement adds a personal touch to these preparations. Assemble baby furniture, pack the hospital bag, and familiarize yourself with the childbirth process. Being prepared ensures you're both ready for the big day.

12. **Strengthening the Bond:** Use this opportunity to make your relationship stronger as a pair. Arrange unique experiences, relish peaceful times together, and honestly discuss your aspirations for the future. Strengthening your relationship during pregnancy sets a positive foundation for the challenges and joys of parenthood.

13. **Balancing Work and Family:** Consider the balance between work and family life. Discuss parental leave options with your employer, and be prepared to adjust your schedule when the baby arrives. Planning ahead ensures you can be present for your partner and child during this critical time.

14. **Educating Yourself:** Continuously educate yourself about pregnancy, childbirth, and parenting. Books, online resources, and support groups provide a wealth of information. Being well-informed equips you to make decisions together, fostering a collaborative and supportive parenting environment.

15. **Cultivating Patience and Understanding:** Above all, cultivate patience and understanding. Pregnancy can be challenging, and every expectant mother's

experience is unique. Be patient with your partner's changing moods and needs, and be understanding of the physical and emotional challenges she faces.

In embracing your role as an expectant father, you are not only preparing for the arrival of your child but also nurturing a strong foundation for your family. Your love, support, and active involvement are the cornerstones of a healthy, happy, and harmonious family life. Welcome to the incredible journey of fatherhood – your presence and dedication make all the difference.

The Emotional Rollercoaster

Pregnancy is a transformative experience, not just for expectant mothers but also for fathers-to-be. While the physical changes and challenges of pregnancy are apparent, the emotional journey is often less discussed but equally significant. Expectant fathers often find themselves on an emotional rollercoaster, navigating a wide range of feelings and uncertainties as they prepare for parenthood.

1. **Excitement and Anticipation:** The journey begins with excitement and anticipation. The positive pregnancy test, the first ultrasound image, and the knowledge that you're going to be a parent fill you with immense joy. The prospect of welcoming a new life into the world is exhilarating, and your dreams for your growing family take shape.

2. **Anxiety and Uncertainty:** However, this excitement can quickly give way to anxiety and uncertainty. You may worry about your partner's health, the baby's well-being, and your ability to be a good parent. These doubts are entirely normal and shared by expectant fathers around the world. Remind yourself that you are not alone in your worries and that it is acceptable to have concerns.

3. **Empathy and Support:** As your partner's body undergoes significant changes, you may find yourself experiencing heightened empathy. Witnessing her physical discomfort or emotional swings can trigger strong feelings of empathy and a desire

to provide support. This is a crucial emotional response that strengthens your bond and ensures her well-being.

4. **Fear and Responsibility:** The realization that you're about to become a father can also bring about fear and a sense of overwhelming responsibility. You may worry about being a provider, protector, and role model. Your desire to be the best father you can be may be strongly influenced by these anxieties.

5. **Joy and Connection:** Despite the emotional rollercoaster, there are times when you just feel happy and connected. Feeling the baby's first kicks, hearing the heartbeat, and seeing the ultrasound images can be profoundly moving experiences. These moments remind you of the incredible journey you're on and the love you already have for your unborn child.

6. **Frustration and Helplessness:** Pregnancy may also present moments of frustration and helplessness. There might be times when you can't alleviate your partner's discomfort or when you're unsure how to respond to her changing needs. Remember that simply being there and offering your support is often enough.

7. **Bonding and Preparation:** Use this time to bond with your partner and prepare for the baby's arrival. Attend prenatal classes together, plan for the nursery, and discuss parenting philosophies. Being ready for motherhood might make you both feel more connected and self-assured.

8. **Handling Relationship Shifts:** Being pregnant may cause changes in your relationship with your spouse. Communication is key to navigating these changes successfully. Communicate honestly about your thoughts, feelings, and worries. Together, you can adapt to the evolving dynamics of your relationship and emerge stronger as a couple.

9. **Finding Support:** Do not be afraid to reach out for assistance from loved ones, friends, or support groups. Sharing your experiences with fellow expectant fathers

can offer comfort and provide valuable insights. Remember that many fathers have been through this emotional rollercoaster before and can offer guidance and reassurance.

10. **Embracing the Journey:** In the end, remember to embrace the journey. The emotional rollercoaster you're on is a natural part of the transition to parenthood. Each twist and turn, every high and low, contributes to your growth as a father and strengthens your connection with your partner.

Your emotions, though sometimes turbulent, reflect your deep commitment to your growing family. By acknowledging and embracing the emotional rollercoaster of pregnancy, you're better equipped to provide the love and support that your partner and child need. Being a parent is an emotional journey with many highs and lows, and this is only the beginning.

Your Unique Perspective

Being a father-to-be is a special and very intimate experience. While you may not be carrying the baby physically, your role is pivotal, and your perspective is entirely your own. Embracing this uniqueness can not only enhance your connection with your partner but also enrich your journey toward parenthood.

Observing Physical Changes

One of the distinctive aspects of your perspective is observing the physical changes in your partner. Witnessing her body transform to accommodate the growing life inside her can be awe-inspiring. From the subtle curve of her belly to the radiant glow on her face, these changes symbolize the miracle of life and your role in bringing it into the world.

Building a Bond

Your bond with the baby begins in a way that's different from your partner's. While she experiences the kicks and hiccups from the inside, your bond develops through touch, talking, and singing. Placing your hand on her belly to feel the baby move establishes a connection that, while different, is just as profound.

Overcoming Challenges Together

Pregnancy often presents challenges, be it emotional, physical, or logistical. Your perspective equips you to tackle these challenges as a team. Whether it's accompanying her to late-night cravings runs or supporting her during moments of exhaustion, your partnership strengthens as you face these hurdles together, setting the stage for your teamwork as parents.

Reflecting on Fatherhood

As an expectant father, you have the opportunity to reflect on what fatherhood means to you. Your unique perspective allows you to contemplate the kind of parent you want to be and the values you want to instill in your child. This exercise in self-reflection can help you grow personally and get ready for the joys and responsibilities of becoming a parent.

Encouraging Independence and Empowerment

Your support can empower your partner in ways that are truly special. Encouraging her to voice her preferences during medical appointments, birthing plans, and parenting decisions fosters a sense of agency and confidence. Your belief in her capabilities strengthens her resolve, creating a positive environment for both her and the baby.

Sharing the Joy of Preparation

Preparing for the baby's arrival is a shared adventure, filled with joy and anticipation. From assembling cribs to selecting baby names, these moments of preparation deepen your connection with both your partner and the baby. Your unique perspective shapes the way you approach these tasks, making them meaningful and memorable.

Embracing the Emotional Impact

Your emotions, often a blend of excitement, nervousness, and profound love, are a testament to your commitment to fatherhood. Embracing these emotions and sharing them with your partner strengthens your relationship. Open communication about your fears and hopes allows both of you to navigate the emotional rollercoaster together, reinforcing your bond.

Preparing for the New Chapter

As the due date approaches, your unique perspective equips you to prepare for the new chapter in your life. You may find yourself contemplating your own childhood, thinking about the lessons you want to pass down, and envisioning the memories you'll create together. Accepting these ideas aids in your mental and emotional preparation for the life-changing experience that is ahead.

Finding Joy in the Everyday Moments

Amidst the preparations and challenges, find joy in the everyday moments. A shared smile, a tender touch, or a heartfelt conversation can bring immense happiness. These moments, unique to your relationship, form the foundation of your family's story, reminding you of the love that binds you together.

Celebrating Your Role

Lastly, celebrate your role as an expectant father. Recognize the significance of your presence, your love, and your support. Your unique perspective enriches the experience for your partner and contributes to the nurturing environment in which your child will grow. Embrace this journey with pride, knowing that your role is indispensable and your love is immeasurable.

Chapter 2:

Preparing for Pregnancy

Establishing a Supportive Environment

Creating a supportive environment during pregnancy is essential for both the expectant mother and father. It not only makes the whole experience better, but it also creates the groundwork for a happy, healthy, and cohesive family. Here's how you can establish a supportive environment for your partner and yourself as you navigate the beautiful journey to parenthood.

1. **Open Communication:** The foundation of a helpful relationship is effective communication. Encourage your partner to talk to you honestly about her wants, worries, and feelings. Be willing to listen without judgment and share your thoughts openly. Honest conversations create an atmosphere of trust and emotional intimacy, fostering a strong bond between both of you.

2. **Empathy and Understanding:** Empathy involves the skill to both comprehend and share in the feelings of someone else. Put yourself in your partner's shoes, recognizing the physical and emotional challenges she faces. Understand that pregnancy can be overwhelming, and her moods might fluctuate. Your understanding and patience can significantly ease her stress and create a nurturing environment.

3. **Active Participation:** Participate actively in every aspect of pregnancy. Attend doctor's appointments, childbirth classes, and parenting workshops together. Being involved in these activities not only educates you both but also strengthens your

sense of partnership. Your active participation shows your commitment and support, making the journey less daunting for both of you.

4. **Emotional Availability:** Be emotionally available and present. Pregnancy can bring up various emotions, from joy and excitement to anxiety and fear. Being emotionally available allows your partner to express her feelings without reservation. Your reassurance and presence during both the highs and lows provide immeasurable comfort.

5. **Promote Self-Care:** Promote Self-Care: Motivate your significant other to give self-care first priority. Pregnancy can be physically taxing, so ensure she gets ample rest, eats nutritious meals, and engages in gentle exercise. Offer to help with home tasks so she can unwind and concentrate on her health. Small gestures like a foot massage or preparing her favorite meal can make a significant difference.

6. **Manage Stress Together:** Stress is a natural part of life, but during pregnancy, it's essential to manage it effectively. Work together to identify stressors and find healthy coping mechanisms. This might include practicing relaxation techniques, taking nature walks, or enjoying hobbies together. You may establish a peaceful and quiet atmosphere at home by controlling stress together.

7. **Nurture Intimacy:** Physical intimacy is a vital aspect of any romantic relationship. During pregnancy, intimacy might change, and it's crucial to adapt together. Communicate openly about your desires and concerns. Emotional intimacy, expressed through affection, cuddling, and kind words, can be just as fulfilling and helps maintain your connection.

8. **Make Plans for the Future:** Making plans for the future helps allay fears of the unknown. Discuss your parenting styles, financial plans, and long-term goals. Together, developing a roadmap offers stability and security. It's also an opportunity to dream about the life you'll build as a family, fostering excitement for the future.

9. **Seek Support Networks:** Do not be afraid to ask for help from members of your family, close friends, or community organizations. Making connections with other pregnant parents can offer insightful conversations and a feeling of belonging. v.

10. **Exercise thankfulness:** Despite the difficulties and planning, express your thankfulness for the pregnancy experience. Each moment, from feeling the baby kick to planning for the nursery, is a precious memory in the making. Acknowledge and appreciate these moments, savoring the anticipation of the new life you're bringing into the world.

Establishing a supportive environment during pregnancy not only benefits your partner but also strengthens your relationship as a couple. Your love, understanding, and active involvement create a nurturing space where both your partner and the baby can thrive.

The Importance of Communication

Any relationship needs communication to survive, but during pregnancy it becomes even more essential. In addition to fortifying the relationship, good communication between partners is essential for navigating the complexity and difficulties of this time of transition. Here's why open, honest, and respectful communication is paramount during pregnancy.

1. **Strengthening Emotional Bonds:** Pregnancy is a rollercoaster of emotions for both partners. By being honest with one another about your aspirations, worries, and expectations, you establish a safe zone. Sharing these feelings strengthens your emotional bond, providing reassurance and understanding during moments of vulnerability. This emotional closeness lays a foundation of trust and support vital for the journey ahead.

2. **Building a Unified Parenting Vision:** Discussing your beliefs, values, and parenting philosophies is essential. Each partner brings their unique perspective, and talking openly about your expectations for parenting can prevent misunderstandings in the future. Agreeing on important aspects such as discipline,

education, and family traditions fosters a unified approach, ensuring consistency and harmony in your child's upbringing.

3. **Addressing Concerns and Anxieties:** Pregnancy comes with its share of worries and anxieties, whether they relate to the baby's health, childbirth, or the challenges of parenthood. Both spouses can express their worries when there is open communication. By addressing these worries together, you can provide mutual reassurance and explore solutions. This shared burden lightens the emotional load, making the journey less overwhelming.

4. **Fostering Physical and Emotional Intimacy:** Pregnancy can alter physical intimacy, and open communication about desires and concerns in this area is essential. Many expectant couples find that emotional intimacy deepens during this period. By talking openly about your changing desires and needs, you can nurture your physical relationship, ensuring that both partners feel loved, desired, and respected.

5. **Making Informed Decisions:** Pregnancy comes with a multitude of decisions, from choosing healthcare providers to planning for the baby's arrival. A mutually beneficial relationship is ensured via effective communication. Making choices that are consistent with your values and aspirations empowers you as parents when you freely discuss possibilities and preferences.

6. **Enhancing Support Systems:** Open communication allows you to express your needs and expectations regarding support from family and friends. Discuss how you want to handle visitors, what kind of help you might need, and what boundaries are important to both of you. Being on the same page ensures that your support system is truly supportive and respectful of your wishes.

7. **Handling Relationship Challenges:** Pregnancy can strain even the strongest relationships due to the stress and changes it brings. The secret to conquering

obstacles is effective communication. By addressing issues promptly and honestly, you can prevent misunderstandings from escalating. Seek support from therapists or counselors if needed; their guidance can facilitate productive communication and help you navigate relationship challenges.

8. **Preparing for the Arrival of Your Baby:** Discussing practical aspects like baby names, nursery arrangements, and birth plans fosters a sense of shared anticipation. It also allows both partners to contribute ideas and feel involved in the preparations. This shared excitement creates a positive atmosphere, making the countdown to the baby's arrival a joyful, collaborative experience.

9. **Encouraging Emotional Expression:** Encourage your partner to express her emotions openly. Pregnancy can bring intense feelings, and having a partner who listens without judgment provides immense comfort. Similarly, express your own emotions and concerns. Vulnerability in communication fosters a deep sense of understanding and emotional intimacy.

10. **Strengthening the Foundation for Parenthood:** Good communication throughout your pregnancy creates a strong foundation for your new role as a parent. It teaches you how to navigate challenges together, fostering resilience and unity. The skills you develop during this time will serve as a cornerstone for your parenting journey, ensuring that you approach the challenges and joys of parenthood as a united team.

In essence, communication during pregnancy is not just about exchanging words; it's about building a bridge of understanding, empathy, and trust between partners. By nurturing this connection, you create a nurturing environment not only for yourselves but also for the little one on the way. Embrace open communication, and you'll find that it not only strengthens your relationship but also enriches your shared experience of parenthood.

Emotional Support for Your Partner

Providing emotional support during this journey can strengthen your relationship and help ease the ups and downs that come with expecting a child. Here are some ways to offer emotional support to your partner during pregnancy.

1. **Be a Good Listener:** One of the best ways to offer emotional support is to listen. Invite your significant other to express her feelings, worries, and thoughts. Establish a space that is judgment-free and safe so she can express herself without fear. Sometimes emotional stress can be reduced by simply being heard.

2. **Validate Her Feelings:** Validation is key to emotional support. Acknowledge your partner's emotions and reassure her that her feelings are valid. For example, if she's feeling anxious about childbirth, you can say, "I understand that you're worried, and it's perfectly normal to feel that way. We'll face this together."

3. **Show Empathy:** Empathy involves understanding and sharing your partner's emotions. Put yourself in her shoes and try to feel what she's feeling. This emotional connection can help her feel understood and less alone in her experiences.

4. **Be Patient:** Pregnancy can bring mood swings and emotional fluctuations. Be patient when your partner experiences these changes. Recognize that she is going through physical and hormonal changes, not you. Your patience can be a soothing balm during these moments.

5. **Offer Physical Affection:** Hugs, cuddles, and handshakes are examples of physical affection that can bring consolation. Physical touch releases feel-good hormones, reducing stress and anxiety. Be attuned to your partner's cues and offer affection when she needs it.

6. **Educate Yourself:** Spend some time learning about pregnancy and the potential emotional difficulties it presents. Being aware of your partner's experiences can

enable you to support them more effectively. Read aloud to her, go to parenting seminars, and discuss her experiences with her.

7. **Share the Experience:** Engage actively in the pregnancy journey. Attend prenatal appointments and ultrasounds together, and ask questions to learn more about the progress of the pregnancy. Sharing these experiences reinforces the idea that you're in this journey together.

8. **Be Flexible:** Pregnancy might lead to unforeseen difficulties like exhaustion or morning sickness. Be adaptable with your plans and her demands. Taking on additional duties or modifying your schedule can occasionally be quite helpful in offering emotional support.

9. **Offer Encouragement:** Positive remarks have great power. Remind your partner of her strength and resilience. Express your pride in her and your gratitude for all of her hard work. Encouragement can boost her confidence and emotional well-being.

10. **Help Reduce Stress:** Take on some of the everyday responsibilities to help reduce her stress. Offer to cook, do the laundry, or run errands to give her more time to rest and relax. A stress-free environment can positively impact her emotional state.

11. **Plan Quality Time:** Set aside quality time for just the two of you. Go for walks, have a date night, or simply spend an evening talking and connecting. These times spent together might deepen your emotional connection.

12. **Anticipate Her Needs:** Pay attention to your partner's needs and anticipate them when possible. For instance, if she's feeling tired, suggest she takes a nap while you handle chores. Small gestures like this show that you're attentive and supportive.

13. **Encourage Self-Care:** Promote self-care for your partner. Encourage her to take time for herself, whether it's a relaxing bath, a hobby she enjoys, or spending time

with friends. Supporting her self-care routine shows that you prioritize her well-being.

14. **Be Reassuring:** Offer reassurance during moments of doubt or worry. Remind your partner that you're there for her no matter what challenges arise. Let her know that you believe in her abilities as a mother.

15. **Seek Assistance Together:** Take into account going to counseling or support groups with your partner. Sometimes, finding other people who have gone through the same things you are and talking to them about your experiences can provide both solace and vital new views.

Remember that emotional support is an ongoing process throughout pregnancy and beyond. Each day brings new emotions and challenges, and your consistent support will be a source of strength for your partner.

Preconception Health and Lifestyle

Preparing for parenthood begins long before your partner becomes pregnant. As an expectant father, your preconception health and lifestyle play a significant role in ensuring a smooth and healthy pregnancy journey for both your partner and your future child. This article will explain the significance of preconception health and show you how to make healthy adjustments.

1. **Recognize the Significance of Preconception Health:** The journey to parenthood starts long before your partner becomes pregnant. Preconception health for both partners significantly influences the health of your baby and the overall pregnancy experience. It's a proactive strategy to guarantee your child has the finest start possible.

2. **Cultivate a Healthy Lifestyle:** Begin by embracing a healthy lifestyle. Eat a diet rich in fruits, vegetables, healthy grains, and lean proteins to ensure balance. Limit

the amount of processed meals, sweetened beverages, and excessive caffeine you consume. Preserving a healthy weight is critical for fertility and the overall health of your partner and future child.

3. **Prioritize Regular Exercise:** Maintaining a healthy body requires regular physical activity. Exercise frequently to improve your fitness and lower your stress levels. However, avoid overexertion or intense exercise that could potentially hinder fertility. Work with a healthcare professional to create an exercise program that suits your needs.

4. **Manage Stress Effectively:** Stress can exert a substantial influence on both fertility and overall well-being. Seek healthy ways to deal with your stress, like engaging in relaxing activities, cultivating a more attentive state of mind, or participating in hobbies that bring you pleasure. Supporting your partner in her stress management is equally vital for her preconception health.

5. **Give Up Smoking:** One of the most important things you can do for your preconception health is to give up smoking. Smoking can diminish fertility, elevate the risk of birth defects, and lead to complications during pregnancy. Seek out support and resources to quit smoking for the sake of your partner and the health of your future child.

6. **Limit Alcohol Consumption:** Drinking too much alcohol might impair fertility and increase the chance of birth abnormalities. While it's not necessary to abstain entirely, it's advisable to limit your alcohol intake to moderate levels or consider abstaining completely while trying to conceive.

7. **Discuss Medications and Supplements:** Have an open discussion with your healthcare provider regarding the medications or supplements you are presently using. Knowing the possible effects of certain drugs on fertility and pregnancy is crucial. Your healthcare provider can offer guidance on any necessary adjustments.

8. **Ensure Immunization:** Make certain that both you and your partner are up to date on vaccinations. Some infections can pose a risk during pregnancy, and maintaining immunity can safeguard both your partner and the baby. To ensure that your immunizations are up to date, speak with your healthcare provider.

9. **Learn About Your Family's Medical History:** This can provide you important information about any genetic or inherited disorders that may impact your child. To identify any possible hazards and make appropriate plans, have discussions with your spouse and healthcare provider.

10. **Support Your Partner's Preconception Health:** Preconception health is a shared responsibility. Encourage and support your partner in making healthy lifestyle choices. You can collaborate as a group to increase the likelihood of a successful pregnancy.

11. **Practice Safe Sex:** If you are not actively attempting to conceive, it's important to maintain safe sex practices to prevent unintended pregnancies. You can consult a healthcare provider to explore contraceptive options that best suit both you and your partner.

12. **Plan Financially:** Being a parent involves financial obligations. Evaluate your financial status and budget for the costs of becoming pregnant, giving birth, and raising a child. Financial stress can be lessened by making a budget and setting aside money for certain expenses.

13. **Educate Yourself:** Lastly, educate yourself about pregnancy, childbirth, and parenting. Reading books, participating in parenting classes, and engaging in open conversations with your partner will help both of you feel more prepared for this life-altering journey.

Chapter 3:

The First Trimester

Pregnancy's first trimester is an amazing experience that is full of changes, obstacles, and joy. Being a father-to-be, you are a crucial component of this experience. In this chapter, we will delve into the various aspects of the first trimester, sharing the unique experiences, discoveries, and strategies to support your partner during this crucial phase.

Sharing the Experience

The moment you learn that you're going to be a father marks the beginning of a life-altering journey. While it's your partner's body undergoing the physical changes of pregnancy, your role as an expectant father is just as crucial. Your love, support, and presence set the stage for a happy and successful pregnancy.

You'll soon discover that your involvement in this voyage extends beyond simply being a bystander. You are a co-pilot, navigating the uncharted waters of pregnancy alongside your partner. Your involvement, engagement, and emotional support are invaluable not only to her but also to the well-being of your future child.

Open Communication

From the very moment you discover the pregnancy, open communication becomes your lifeline. Honest and transparent conversations with your partner about her feelings, hopes, and expectations are vital. This is your chance to express your excitement to each other and to talk about any worries or fears.

Good communication is essential to a solid and encouraging collaboration. It fosters an atmosphere of trust and safety where both partners feel comfortable sharing their feelings, fears, and goals. By sharing your thoughts openly, you strengthen the emotional bond between you and set a precedent for the open dialogue that will serve as the bedrock of your relationship as parents.

Becoming a Team

Parenthood is a team effort, and the first trimester is the beginning of your shared journey. Embrace your role as a team, where both partners actively participate in the decision-making process and work together toward common goals.

This is a time to discuss and establish your shared vision for parenthood. It involves exploring your values, parenting styles, and future aspirations. A harmonious and cohesive approach to parenting requires that parents communicate clearly and establish common ground. When you function as a team, you become each other's greatest allies in the adventures and challenges that lie ahead.

Discovering the Pregnancy

The moment you discover that you're going to be parents is a milestone that you'll remember for the rest of your lives. Whether it happens with the appearance of those two pink lines on a home pregnancy test or through a more elaborate announcement, it's a moment filled with awe and wonder.

The Positive Test

The first tangible sign of pregnancy often comes with a home pregnancy test. When the test results are good, an exciting and life-changing adventure begins. You might feel a range of feelings, such as intense delight or a deep sense of duty. Expectant fathers everywhere experience these feelings, which attests to the importance of the occasion.

Managing Emotions

Alongside the joy of the positive test, you and your partner may also experience a range of other emotions. Nervousness, anxiety, and even a touch of fear are entirely natural reactions. The prospect of becoming parents is life-altering, and it's entirely reasonable to feel a mixture of excitement and trepidation.

The key to managing these emotions is open and empathetic communication. Express your emotions openly with your partner, and support her in sharing her feelings as well. Acknowledge each other's emotions without judgment, and remember that you are in this together. Your emotional support for each other during this period is invaluable and lays the foundation for the teamwork that will carry you through parenthood.

Sharing the News

The decision of when and how to share the news of your pregnancy with family and friends is a personal one. Some couples choose to keep the news to themselves during the first trimester, while others are eager to share their joy with loved ones right away.

It's crucial to take your partner's preferences and any prevailing cultural or familial customs into account when deciding when to make the announcement. Some couples choose to share the news earlier with close family members and friends and wait until after the first trimester to make a broader announcement, as this is when the risk of miscarriage typically decreases.

In either case, sharing the news of your pregnancy is an opportunity to celebrate this milestone with loved ones. Their support and excitement can be a source of great joy and encouragement for both you and your partner.

Dealing with Hormonal Changes

Hormonal changes are a hallmark of the first trimester of pregnancy. These shifts are not only responsible for the physical changes your partner experiences but also influence her emotional state. As an expectant father, it's vital to understand these hormonal changes and their impact on your partner's well-being.

Hormone levels spike during the first trimester, particularly progesterone and human chorionic gonadotropin (hCG). These hormones play a vital role in sustaining the pregnancy, yet they can also give rise to various physical and emotional symptoms.

Your role in providing emotional support to your partner during this phase cannot be overstated. The emotional well-being of expectant mothers is intrinsically tied to their overall health and the health of the baby.

As hormonal changes bring about mood swings, increased sensitivity, and heightened emotions, your presence as a steady and supportive partner becomes paramount Here's how to provide emotional support:

1. **Empathy:** Try to put yourself in your partner's position and comprehend her thoughts, emotions, and experiences. Being able to relate to someone else's emotions is called empathy. By showing empathy, you create a deeper connection and demonstrate that you are there to support her, no matter how intense her emotions may be.

2. **Active Listening:** Sometimes, all your partner needs is someone to listen without judgment or offering solutions. As you actively listen to her, provide a secure environment in which she can share her ideas and emotions. Encourage her to share her joys, concerns, and fears.

3. **Reassurance:** Remind your girlfriend that you will always be there for her. Offer words of reassurance and comfort during moments of doubt or anxiety. Tell her you are her dependable companion and that you are confident she can complete this journey.

4. **Affection:** Physical affection can be incredibly comforting during times of emotional upheaval. Without using words, love and support can be expressed with a simple embrace, gentle touch, or cuddle.

5. **Patience:** Understand that hormonal changes can lead to mood swings and varying emotional states. Exercise patience and refrain from taking any emotional outbursts personally. Instead, focus on being a calming presence and a source of stability.

6. **Encouragement:** Encourage your partner to express her emotions openly. Repressing emotions can make you more stressed and anxious. Tell her it's all OK to share her highs and lows with you.

7. **Engage in Self-Care:** Maintaining one's emotional health requires self-care. Encourage and assist your significant other to engage in enjoyable and calming activities. Whether it's a warm bath, a leisurely walk, or indulging in a hobby, supporting her self-care routine demonstrates your commitment to her emotional health.

8. **Seek Professional Help if Needed:** In some cases, hormonal changes can lead to more profound emotional challenges, such as depression or anxiety. If you notice persistent and severe emotional distress in your partner, consider seeking the guidance of a mental health professional or counselor. Your partner's well-being should always be the top priority.

Managing Morning Sickness

Morning sickness is one of the most prevalent pregnancy symptoms during the first trimester. It can happen at any time of day, despite its name. Your partner may experience a range of symptoms, including nausea, vomiting, food aversions, and heightened sensitivity to certain smells.

Even while feeling ill in the morning during pregnancy is typically viewed as a good indicator that the pregnancy is going well, it might prove difficult to handle. As an expectant father, it's important to be prepared for these potential challenges and to support your partner through them.

Helping your significant other deal with morning sickness will make her feel much more comfortable and in better health. Here are some strategies to consider:

1. **Prepare Simple Meals:** Cook light, easily digestible meals for your partner. Opt for bland foods like crackers, rice, or toast, which can often alleviate nausea. Avoid heavy, greasy, or strongly flavored dishes.

2. **Ginger:** Ginger The anti-nausea effects of ginger are well-known. Keep ginger candies, ginger tea, or ginger ale on hand for your partner to sip or chew when she's feeling nauseous.

3. **Remain Hydrated:** The symptoms of morning sickness can worsen if you're dehydrated. Throughout the day, remind your companion to stay hydrated by having water, clear liquids, or electrolyte drinks. Ice chips or popsicles can also help maintain fluid balance.

4. **Regular, Small Meals:** Instead of having three substantial meals throughout the day, advise your companion to eat frequently, small meals. Sometimes, feeling sick to oneself makes sickness worse.

5. **Vitamin B6:** With your healthcare provider's approval, consider supplementing with vitamin B6, which has been shown to alleviate nausea in some pregnant individuals.

6. **Fresh Air:** Encourage your partner to step outside for some fresh air when she's feeling queasy. At times, a change of surroundings and some fresh air can offer relief.

7. **Acupressure Bands:** Acupressure wristbands designed for morning sickness may help alleviate symptoms. These bracelets apply pressure to particular acupuncture spots, which are thought to lessen nausea.

8. **Avoid Triggers:** Identify any particular smells, foods, or situations that trigger nausea for your partner, and do your best to minimize exposure to these triggers.

9. **Provide Emotional Support:** Morning sickness can be physically and emotionally draining. Offer emotional support, be patient, and reassure your partner that these symptoms are temporary and often a sign of a healthy pregnancy.

10. **Accompany Her to Appointments:** Attend prenatal appointments with your partner. Her healthcare provider can provide guidance on managing morning sickness and may recommend specific interventions if symptoms are severe.

11. **Examine Alternative Therapies:** Acupuncture and hypnosis are two alternative therapies that some people use to treat their morning sickness. Converse with your healthcare provider to assess the safety and suitability of these choices for your partner.

12. **Stay Informed:** Educate yourself about morning sickness and its management. Knowing about the illness will enable you to support your partner more effectively and give wise advice.

Attending Doctor's Appointments

Attending prenatal doctor's appointments is a crucial aspect of supporting your partner during her pregnancy journey. These consultations offer extremely helpful information regarding the development of the pregnancy as a whole, the health of both your partner and your baby, and offer opportunities for you to actively participate in the process.

Why Your Presence Matters

- **Emotional Support:** Pregnancy can be emotionally overwhelming, filled with excitement, anticipation, and sometimes anxiety. Your partner benefits from your emotional support and assurance when you attend doctor's appointments. Knowing that you're by her side during these crucial moments can be comforting and empowering.
- **Information and Understanding:** Prenatal appointments provide an opportunity for both you and your partner to gain a deeper understanding of the

pregnancy. Medical professionals describe the baby's growth, address any possible worries, and provide advice on how to have a good pregnancy. Your active participation allows you to absorb this information firsthand.

- **Shared Decision-Making:** Prenatal care often involves important decisions, such as choosing a birthing plan, discussing prenatal tests, and exploring pain management options. Your involvement in these discussions ensures that both you and your partner have a say in the decisions that affect the pregnancy and birth experience.

Tips for Attending Doctor's Appointments

1. **Be Punctual:** Arrive on time for appointments to respect the healthcare provider's schedule and minimize stress for your partner.

2. **Prepare Questions:** Talk about any queries or worries you both may have before to the appointment. Jot them down so you don't forget during the appointment.

3. **Actively Listen:** Pay close attention to the healthcare provider's explanations and recommendations. Please don't hesitate to ask for clarification if something is unclear.

4. **Offer Comfort:** Holding your partner's hand or providing physical comfort during examinations can be reassuring. Be attentive to her needs and emotions.

5. **Take Notes:** Consider bringing a notebook to jot down important information provided during the appointment. This can help you both remember details discussed.

6. **Ask About Ultrasound:** If an ultrasound is scheduled, inquire if you can be present to see the baby on the monitor. Many expectant fathers find this moment especially meaningful.

7. **Celebrate Milestones:** After each appointment, take a moment to celebrate the baby's progress. Whether it's listening to the baby's heartbeat or discussing ultrasound images, these are moments to cherish.

8. **Plan Future Appointments:** Coordinate your schedules to ensure you can attend as many appointments as possible throughout the pregnancy. Talk to your partner about this and make plans appropriately.

Attending prenatal appointments is just one aspect of creating a supportive environment for your partner during pregnancy. Beyond the doctor's office, continue to be actively involved in the pregnancy journey. Encourage open communication, provide emotional support, and actively participate in decisions regarding prenatal care and childbirth plans.

Your commitment to attending appointments and being an engaged partner demonstrates your dedication to your growing family. It strengthens your partnership and ensures that both you and your partner are well-informed and prepared for the beautiful journey of parenthood that lies ahead.

Chapter 4:

The Second Trimester

The second trimester of pregnancy is a magical time filled with anticipation and hope. As an expectant father, your role during this phase remains indispensable. In this chapter, we'll explore the unique aspects of the second trimester, from being a rock of support for your partner to understanding the physical changes she's going through, preparing for your baby's arrival, gaining insights into ultrasounds, and enrolling in birthing and newborn care classes.

Being the Rock

The second trimester, which typically spans from the 13th to the 27th week of pregnancy, is a unique phase for expectant mothers. It is during this period when many early pregnancy discomforts, such as morning sickness and exhaustion, start to go away. A renewed sense of energy often accompanies the second trimester, making it an ideal time for couples to bond and prepare for parenthood.

However, it's essential to remember that while some discomforts may diminish, the emotional and physical changes your partner experiences continue to shape her pregnancy journey. As her partner, your role in providing emotional support and stability becomes even more critical during this period.

Providing Emotional Support

Pregnancy brings about a whirlwind of emotions for expectant mothers. The initial excitement of discovering the pregnancy is often intertwined with anxieties about labor, the responsibilities of parenthood, and concerns about body image. As her partner, you can be a reassuring presence by creating a safe and empathetic space for her to express these feelings.

Sincere and transparent communication is essential to providing emotional assistance. Invite your significant other to express her hopes, anxieties, and thoughts. Be an active and compassionate listener, and let her know that her emotions are valid, even if they fluctuate from day to day.

It's crucial to maintain patience and understanding during this time. Pregnancy hormones can intensify emotions, and your partner may experience mood swings. Instead of taking these changes personally, remind yourself that it's a natural part of the pregnancy process, and your unwavering support can help ease her emotional rollercoaster.

Celebrating Milestones

The second trimester is a period of notable milestones, one of the most profound being when your partner first feels the baby's movements, known as "quickening." These subtle flutters and kicks are a tangible reminder of the life growing within her, and they offer an excellent opportunity for you to share in the joy of the pregnancy.

To participate in these moments, place your hand gently on her belly and wait for those subtle kicks and movements. This physical connection with your baby is a powerful bonding experience. It reaffirms your commitment to each other and your growing family.

Moreover, these shared experiences strengthen your emotional connection as a couple. They provide opportunities to express your love and excitement for the journey ahead. Together, you will treasure the enduring memories you make when you celebrate these milestones.

Planning Together

It's also time to start making plans for the baby's arrival during the second trimester. Engage in meaningful discussions with your partner about your shared parenting philosophy, baby names, and your vision for the childbirth experience. Collaborating on these decisions strengthens your partnership and establishes a strong foundation for your parenting journey.

Making a birth plan is a crucial step in this procedure. A birth plan outlines your partner's preferences for labor and delivery, covering aspects like pain management, birthing environment, and medical interventions. By discussing and creating this plan together, you ensure that your partner's wishes are considered and respected during the childbirth experience.

Furthermore, this planning process is an opportunity to involve both partners actively. Your support in crafting the birth plan showcases your commitment to being a reliable and involved partner throughout the pregnancy and beyond.

Physical Changes and Comfort Measures

While this trimester typically brings more physical comfort for expectant mothers, it's essential to recognize and understand the changes their bodies undergo during this time. As an expectant father, your role in providing support and comfort measures is crucial in helping your partner navigate this transformative journey.

Body Changes

One of the most apparent physical changes during the second trimester is the noticeable growth of the baby bump. Your partner's silhouette will alter as the uterus grows to fit the growing baby. This can be an exciting and beautiful transformation, but it may also come with some discomfort.

It's critical to recognize and value these developments. Compliment your partner on her pregnancy glow and the remarkable way her body is nurturing your child. Tell her about the amazing journey she's taken and the strength she has.

While some women embrace these body changes, others may feel self-conscious. Remind her that these changes are evidence of the wonder of life and promote body confidence. Offer your unwavering support by being an empathetic and understanding partner.

Breast Changes

In addition to the growing belly, many expectant mothers experience changes in their breasts during the second trimester. The body often experiences breast growth and pain while it gets ready to nurse.

These changes can sometimes be uncomfortable or even painful for your partner. Offer her reassurance and comfort by being mindful of her feelings. Be considerate of her sensitivity and avoid squeezing or touching her breasts without her consent. If she experiences discomfort, suggest wearing a comfortable and supportive bra designed for pregnancy.

Educate yourself about breastfeeding to provide meaningful support when the time comes. Attend breastfeeding classes together, learn about proper latch techniques, and discuss your role in supporting successful breastfeeding. Your proactive participation in this stage of pregnancy can allay worries and make breastfeeding more enjoyable.

Skin Changes

Alterations in Skin Certain women may experience skin changes as the second trimester goes on. Stretch marks are one of the most prevalent skin-related issues that people have. These reddish or purplish streaks often appear on the abdomen, breasts, thighs, and hips as the skin stretches to accommodate the growing baby.

Although many women consider stretch marks to be a normal aspect of pregnancy, they can occasionally cause anxiety or self-consciousness. Assure your partner that these marks are a monument to the amazing journey of parenting and encourage her to accept her changing body.

There is a wide variety of lotions and oils on the market that make the promise that they can reduce the visibility of stretch marks. While their effectiveness can vary, the act of massaging these products onto her skin can be a comforting and bonding experience. Offer to apply these creams for her, turning it into a loving and intimate ritual.

Comfort Measures

To further support your partner's physical comfort during the second trimester, explore various comfort measures together:

1. **Prenatal Yoga:** Consider enrolling in prenatal yoga classes designed specifically for expectant mothers. The goals of these classes are to increase muscular elasticity, decrease tension, and encourage relaxation. Participating as a couple not only enhances your partner's well-being but also provides quality time together.

2. **Prenatal Massages:** Treat your partner to prenatal massages. These specialized massages target areas that may be experiencing discomfort due to pregnancy-related changes. A massage's calming touch can ease tension in the muscles and encourage relaxation.

3. **Pregnancy Pillow:** Purchasing a pregnancy cushion can greatly improve the quality of sleep for your significant other. These specially designed pillows provide essential support for her changing body, facilitating a more comfortable sleeping position. Urge her to experiment with various pillow combinations until she finds the most comfortable one.

4. **Hydration and Nutrition:** Gently emphasize to your partner the significance of staying well-hydrated and sustaining a balanced diet. Offer to prepare nutritious meals together and keep her water bottle filled. She has to drink enough water and eat a healthy diet in order to feel comfortable and be well overall.

By actively participating in these comfort measures and offering unwavering emotional support, you contribute to a positive and enjoyable second trimester for your partner.

Understanding Ultrasound

Ultrasound scans are an integral part of prenatal care during the second trimester. These scans offer invaluable insights into the development and well-being of your baby, allowing you and your partner to establish a deeper connection with your growing child.

Types of Ultrasounds

In the second trimester, you can anticipate several ultrasound scans, each serving a specific purpose. The anatomy scan, typically conducted around the 20-week mark, is one of the most significant. During this scan, healthcare providers meticulously examine your baby's anatomy, checking for any developmental issues or abnormalities.

The gender reveal scan is another common ultrasound in the second trimester, offering you the opportunity to learn your baby's sex if you wish to do so. Additionally, periodic ultrasounds may be conducted to monitor your baby's growth and well-being.

Bonding Opportunity

Ultrasound appointments provide a unique and heartwarming opportunity for both you and your partner to bond with your baby. Witnessing the baby's movements, hearing the rhythmic heartbeat, and observing their growth on the ultrasound screen are profoundly moving experiences.

Take the time to ask questions and seek explanations from the healthcare provider during these appointments. Understanding what you're seeing on the screen enhances your appreciation of these remarkable moments. In order to save your precious pregnancy moments, think about capturing pictures or recording the ultrasound.

Preparing the Home and Nursery

As your partner's pregnancy progresses, the excitement of welcoming your little one into the world grows exponentially. One of the most joyful and tangible ways to prepare for your baby's arrival is by setting up their nursery and ensuring your home is a safe and welcoming environment. Preparing the home and nursery is not just about assembling cribs and choosing colors; it's about creating a haven where your child will thrive and feel loved. Let's explore the essential steps to make your home and nursery a perfect sanctuary for your little one.

Creating a Nursery with Love and Care

1. **Choose a Theme:** Start by selecting a theme or color scheme for the nursery. Whether it's a soothing pastel palette, a vibrant jungle adventure, or a celestial dreamland, the theme sets the tone for the room. Involve your partner in this decision, ensuring the nursery reflects both your styles and preferences.

2. **Furniture and Layout:** Purchase basic nursery furnishings including a changing table, crib, and storage containers. Choose furniture that is safe, secure, long-lasting, and compliant with the most recent safety regulations. Arrange the furniture to create a functional layout, keeping in mind easy access to baby essentials like diapers, wipes, and clothes.

3. **Decorate Thoughtfully:** Personalize the nursery with thoughtful decorations. Consider framed artwork, wall decals, or a growth chart. Integrate elements that hold sentimental value, such as handmade crafts or items gifted by friends and family. This intimate touch makes the ambiance cozy and loving.

4. **Comfortable Nursing Area:** If your partner plans to breastfeed, create a comfortable nursing corner in the nursery. Add a cozy chair or glider with soft cushions, a side table for placing necessities, and soft lighting. This area will become a haven for late-night feeds and quiet bonding moments.

5. **Safety First:** Childproof the nursery meticulously. Make sure the crib slats are spaced correctly, cover electrical outlets, and fasten large furniture to the walls to prevent it from toppling over. If required, install safety gates and window guards. Regularly inspect toys and furnishings for any potential hazards.

6. **Organize Baby Essentials:** Set up the nursery with baby essentials within easy reach. Use labeled baskets or drawers for organizing diapers, wipes, clothing, and blankets. A well-organized nursery simplifies caregiving tasks and creates a serene atmosphere.

Preparing Your Home for the Baby's Arrival

1. **Childproofing Your Home:** Beyond the nursery, assess the entire house for potential hazards. Put in safety gates on both sides of steps. Cover sharp corners of furniture with safety padding. Lock cabinets that hold medicines, cleaning supplies, and other potentially dangerous things. Make sure the infant cannot choke on any little objects or loose cables.

2. **Preparing the Bedroom:** If your baby will be sharing your room initially, consider setting up a bassinet or a crib beside your bed for convenient nighttime care. Make sure you have a changing station with diapers, wipes, and a comfortable changing mat nearby.

3. **Stock Up on Supplies:** Get ready for the baby's arrival by storing necessities including feeding supplies, diapers, wipes, baby outfits, and blankets. Having an ample supply reduces stress in the early days, allowing you to focus on bonding with your newborn.

4. **Learn Baby First Aid:** Enroll in a baby first aid and CPR course. Knowing how to respond to emergencies provides confidence and ensures you can react effectively in critical situations. It's a skill that every parent should possess.

5. **Create a Support System:** Parenthood can be overwhelming, especially in the early days. Create a network of friends, relatives, and other parents to lean on. Being able to turn to others for support, guidance, or just to lend an ear can have a big impact on your parenting journey.

Preparing your home and nursery is a labor of love, symbolizing the anticipation and devotion you have for your little one. By approaching this task with care, attention to detail, and a focus on safety, you're not just setting up a physical space but also creating a foundation of love, security, and warmth.

Birthing and Newborn Care Classes

Education is an invaluable tool as you and your partner prepare for the journey of parenthood. Enrolling in birthing and newborn care classes together can bolster your confidence and equip you with essential knowledge and skills.

Childbirth Education

Birthing classes, also known as childbirth education classes, cover a wide range of topics related to labor and delivery. These classes delve into the various stages of labor, pain management options, relaxation techniques, and the logistics of the childbirth process.

Participating in these classes as a couple offers numerous benefits:

- **Knowledge:** Childbirth education classes provide in-depth information about the birthing process. Knowing what to anticipate throughout labor and delivery makes you and your partner feel more prepared and confident.
- **Bonding:** Co-attending lessons promotes togetherness and shared accountability. It allows you to learn and practice various techniques as a team, creating a deeper connection.
- **Questions and Clarifications:** Classes on childbirth provide participants with a chance to pose questions, receive explanation, and obtain a more in-depth awareness of the process of giving birth. Instructors with experience can provide expert guidance and address any concerns.
- **Tailoring Your Birth Plan:** Armed with knowledge from these classes, you can work with your partner to create a birth plan that aligns with her preferences and comfort. Discuss the type of birthing environment she envisions, her choices for pain management, and any other aspects of labor and delivery.
- **Labor Coach Role:** Learning about pain management techniques and relaxation methods enables you to support your partner effectively during labor. You can become her trusted labor coach, offering encouragement and assistance when needed.

Newborn Care

Newborn care classes offer insights into essential aspects of caring for your baby during the initial weeks and months of their life. Topics covered often include:

1. **Feeding:** Newborn care classes provide guidance on both breastfeeding and bottle-feeding. Both you and your partner can have a more pleasant and pleasurable feeding experience if you are aware of the right techniques, placement, and cues from the baby.

2. **Diapering and Soothing:** You'll learn how to change diapers efficiently and effectively, ensuring your baby stays clean and comfortable. Additionally, classes cover soothing techniques to calm a fussy baby, including swaddling and gentle rocking.

3. **Recognizing Cues:** Understanding your baby's cues is crucial for responsive and attentive parenting. Newborn care classes teach you how to recognize signs of hunger, discomfort, and sleepiness, enabling you to respond promptly to your baby's needs.

4. **Safety:** Infant safety is a top priority. Classes often include essential safety measures such as safe sleep practices, car seat safety, and tips for creating a safe home environment for your newborn.

5. **Basic First Aid:** Consider enrolling in infant CPR and first aid classes as part of your newborn care preparation. Although the need for these skills is infrequent, possessing the knowledge and self-assurance to react to emergencies can be priceless when it comes to ensuring your baby's safety.

Creating a Support Network

In addition to the wealth of information provided, birthing and parenting classes offer another valuable benefit: the opportunity to connect with other expectant parents. Building a support network of friends who are experiencing similar milestones can be incredibly reassuring and informative.

A sense of camaraderie is fostered by sharing your experiences, exchanging parenting advice, and providing support to one another. Parenthood may present its challenges along the way, but having a circle of friends who comprehend and empathize with your joys and worries can amplify the fulfillment of the journey.

Chapter 5:

The Third Trimester

The third trimester is the last stage of the gestational cycle. With the due date approaching, the countdown to meeting your baby begins in earnest. This trimester is filled with anticipation, preparations, and, of course, the excitement of finally holding your little one in your arms.

The Countdown Begins

As the third trimester unfolds, one of the most captivating aspects is the increasing awareness of your baby's presence. You may find that you can feel the baby's movements more distinctly, as their kicks, rolls, and wiggles become stronger and more frequent. Encourage your partner to take joy in these moments, as they provide a tangible connection between you, your baby, and the journey you are embarking on together.

A wonderful way to bond during this time is by monitoring the baby's kick count. Counting the baby's movements is a straightforward but useful technique to make sure they are active and healthy. Healthcare providers often recommend monitoring kick counts regularly during the third trimester. This practice not only offers peace of mind but also strengthens the bond between you, your partner, and your growing baby.

Attending Prenatal Checkups Together

Throughout the third trimester, your partner will continue to have regular prenatal checkups with her healthcare provider. The closer the deadline gets, the more often these appointments occur. Attending these checkups with your partner is a wonderful way to stay informed about the baby's progress and receive any necessary guidance.

By attending these sessions, you may be a proactive and encouraging partner. You have the opportunity to inquire, seek explanation, and obtain a more in-depth knowledge of the growth of the baby. Additionally, it's a chance to see ultrasound pictures, hear the baby's heartbeat, and observe the amazing changes occurring.

Your presence at these appointments demonstrates your commitment to being an engaged and involved partner in this journey. It's a chance to share in the excitement of monitoring your baby's health and growth and to provide comfort and reassurance to your partner.

Breathing Exercises and Pelvic Floor Exercises

As the due date approaches, preparing for labor and birth becomes a focal point. Motivate your partner to participate in activities that enhance both physical and mental preparedness for labor. Exercises for the pelvic floor and breathing are two crucial activities for the third trimester.

1. **Breathing Exercises:** Deep breathing exercises are a valuable tool for managing stress and anxiety during pregnancy. They can also be incredibly beneficial during labor. Encourage your partner to practice deep breathing techniques regularly. These exercises not only help with relaxation but also enhance oxygen flow, which is crucial for both mother and baby.

2. **Pelvic Floor Exercises:** Engaging in pelvic floor exercises, commonly identified as Kegels, is vital for preparing the pelvic muscles for labor and facilitating postpartum recovery. These activities assist in strengthening the muscles which bolster the bladder, as well as those that maintain the uterus and the colon. Consistent practice can result in enhanced muscle tone and improved control during the labor and childbirth process.

Engaging in these exercises together can be a bonding experience. You can join your partner in practicing deep breathing techniques, and she can include you in her pelvic floor exercise routine. Engaging in these exercises enhances not only your physical readiness but also your couple's emotional bond.

Braxton Hicks Contractions

As the third trimester advances, you may experience Braxton Hicks contractions, commonly known as "practice contractions." These contractions are a typical part of pregnancy that help get the body ready for labor. Although they can be uncomfortable, they are typically not painful and are not the same as actual labor contractions.

Braxton Hicks contractions tend to be irregular, less intense, and shorter in duration compared to true labor contractions. They often come and go without a discernible pattern. These contractions can cause anxiety in some expectant parents, particularly in first-time mothers. That being said, it's critical to recognize that Braxton Hicks contractions are a typical aspect of pregnancy.

Coping with Braxton Hicks Contractions

As an expectant father, you can play a vital role in helping your partner cope with Braxton Hicks contractions:

1. **Provide Support:** Offer emotional support and reassurance to your partner. Remind her that Braxton Hicks contractions are a normal part of pregnancy and not a cause for alarm. Your calm and comforting presence can ease her anxiety.

2. **Encourage Hydration:** Staying well-hydrated can help alleviate Braxton Hicks contractions. Urge your significant other to stay hydrated throughout the day. Dehydration can make these contractions more frequent and uncomfortable.

3. **Rest and Change Positions:** If your partner is experiencing Braxton Hicks contractions, suggest that she take a break and rest. Switching positions, reclining on her left side, or enjoying a warm bath can assist in alleviating discomfort.

4. **Monitor Frequency:** While Braxton Hicks contractions are typically irregular, you can help your partner monitor their frequency and duration. If they become more frequent or painful, it's a good idea to contact her healthcare provider for guidance.

5. **Distraction:** Sometimes, engaging in a distracting activity can help take your partner's mind off the contractions. Watching a movie, practicing relaxation techniques, or going for a short walk can be effective distractions.

6. **Preparation for Labor:** Use these practice contractions as an opportunity to prepare for labor. Encourage your partner to practice relaxation and breathing techniques, which will be valuable during actual labor.

As mentioned earlier, Braxton Hicks contractions are a normal and necessary part of pregnancy. They may cause discomfort, but they may not necessarily indicate that labor will soon begin. However, if your partner experiences contractions that are regular, become increasingly painful, or are accompanied by other symptoms such as bleeding or a decrease in fetal movement, it's crucial to contact her healthcare provider promptly.

Baby Shower Planning

Baby showers are a cherished tradition that allows friends and family to come together and celebrate the impending arrival of your little one. Planning a baby shower is a special way to mark this joyous occasion and create lasting memories. Here's how you can approach the planning process:

1. **Date and Venue:** The initial step in planning a baby shower is to decide on a date and venue. Think about where you would like to have the party: at your house, at a relative's house, or at a rental place. Ensure the date aligns with your partner's availability and comfort.

2. **Guest List:** Make a guest list with your closest and most loved friends and relatives. Consult with your partner to ensure all essential people are invited, and consider any special preferences or traditions that you both may have regarding the guest list.

3. **Theme and Decorations:** Choose a theme or color scheme for the baby shower. The chosen theme establishes the ambiance for the occasion and can draw inspiration from your personal interests, hobbies, or the decor of the baby's nursery. Banners, balloons, and table settings are examples of decorations that can express the selected theme and create a joyous environment.

4. **Games and Activities:** Arrange enjoyable games and activities to ensure that your guests remain engaged and entertained. Popular options include guessing the baby's birthdate and playing baby-themed bingo. Together with your closest and most cherished friends and family, create a guest list.

5. **Gift Registry:** Create a gift registry to guide guests in choosing presents. Incorporate a diverse range of items, including baby clothing, diapers, infant equipment, and essential nursery items. A well-organized gift registry ensures that your baby receives items that are practical and useful.

The baby shower is a chance for friends and family to express their love and support in addition to celebrating your growing family. It's a time to share in the joy of parenthood and receive blessings and well-wishes from those who care about you and your baby.

The Role of a Co-Ed Baby Shower

Traditionally, baby showers have been predominantly attended by women, with the focus centered on the expectant mother. However, in recent years, co-ed baby showers, where both men and women are invited, have gained popularity. These gatherings emphasize the celebration of parenthood as a shared journey and provide a unique opportunity for both partners to come together, celebrate, and seek support from their loved ones.

Co-ed baby showers challenge traditional gender norms and expectations by inviting both partners to be active participants in the celebration. They represent a shift toward a more egalitarian approach to parenthood, where both parents are equally involved and supported throughout the journey.

Inclusivity for All

One of the key advantages of co-ed baby showers is inclusivity. By inviting both men and women, you create an environment where all friends and family members can participate and share in the joy of welcoming a new life. This inclusivity helps strengthen relationships, fosters a sense of community, and ensures that both partners feel equally supported and celebrated.

Sharing the Responsibility

Co-ed baby showers reflect the modern reality of shared responsibilities in parenting. They acknowledge that fathers-to-be play a vital role in the journey from pregnancy to parenthood. By including both partners, co-ed baby showers reinforce the idea that parenting is a collaborative effort, and the responsibilities and joys of parenthood are shared equally.

Activities for Everyone

When planning a co-ed baby shower, it's essential to consider activities and games that are enjoyable for everyone, regardless of gender. Instead of traditional baby shower games that may be geared more towards women, opt for games and activities that foster a relaxed and inclusive atmosphere.

Some ideas for co-ed baby shower activities include:

- **Diaper Changing Challenge:** A lighthearted contest between couples to see who can change a doll's diaper the fastest.
- **Baby Food Tasting:** Blindfolded participants taste different baby foods and guess the flavors, creating a fun and amusing experience.
- **Parenting Advice Cards:** Guests, regardless of gender, can share their parenting advice and well-wishes, providing valuable insights and heartfelt messages.

A Chance to Share Feelings and Expectations

Co-ed baby showers provide a platform for both partners to express their feelings, hopes, and expectations for parenthood. You can incorporate moments during the event where each partner shares their thoughts and emotions. These heartfelt exchanges can deepen your connection as a couple and create beautiful memories.

Gifts for Both

In a co-ed baby shower, the gift-giving aspect can also reflect the idea of shared responsibilities. Encourage guests to bring gifts that cater to both parents' needs and preferences. While baby gifts are essential and appreciated, consider items that enhance your life as a couple. This can include items that support your well-being, relaxation, and relationship, as well as practical items for the baby.

Food and Refreshments for All Tastes

When planning the menu for a co-ed baby shower, take into account the tastes and preferences of both men and women. Incorporate a variety of foods and beverages that cater to different dietary choices and ensure that everyone feels comfortable and well-fed. A varied menu contributes to making dining inclusive and pleasurable for all patrons.

Packing the Hospital Bag

Packing the hospital bag is a practical and symbolic task that marks the final stages of pregnancy. It's a tangible reminder that the big day is approaching when you'll welcome your precious baby into the world. A well-prepared hospital bag ensures that you and your partner are fully equipped to navigate the experience of labor and childbirth with comfort and confidence.

Here's a comprehensive checklist of essential items to include in the hospital bag:

For Your Partner

1. **Identification and Hospital Documents:** Ensure that you have all necessary identification, medical records, and hospital admission documents readily available. This includes your partner's ID, insurance information, and any required paperwork from her healthcare provider.

2. **Comfortable Clothing:** Pack a selection of comfortable clothing for your partner. Opt for loose-fitting pajamas, a cozy robe, and comfortable slippers. These items will provide comfort during labor and the postpartum period.

3. **Toiletries:** Provide a basic toiletry kit that includes toothbrushes, toothpaste, shampoo, conditioner, soap, and any other personal hygiene products your significant other may want. Having these familiar items on hand can make a significant difference in her comfort.

4. **Snacks:** Pack some non-perishable snacks for both you and your partner. Labor can be a lengthy process, and having easily accessible snacks can help maintain energy levels.

5. **Entertainment:** To pass the time during labor and the hospital stay, think about bringing novels, periodicals, or electronic gadgets with headphones. Entertainment options that are soothing can be a nice diversion.

6. **Pillow and Blanket:** While the hospital provides bedding, having a familiar pillow and blanket from home can provide added comfort and a sense of familiarity.

For the Baby:

1. **Baby Clothes:** Pack a few sets of newborn clothing for your baby, including onesies, sleepers, and hats. These should be soft and gentle on the baby's delicate skin.

2. **Diapers and Wipes:** Ensure you have a supply of newborn diapers and baby wipes. It's essential to have these items ready for the baby's immediate needs.

3. **Baby Blanket:** Bring a soft and cozy blanket for swaddling and keeping the baby warm. Hospitals may provide some essentials, but having your own blanket can be a comforting touch.

4. **Car Seat:** One of the most critical items to bring is a properly installed infant car seat. It's essential for securely transferring your infant from the hospital to your house. Ensure you understand how to install it correctly, as this is a hospital requirement.

For Both:

1. **Phone and Charger:** Keep your phone and charger handy to stay in touch with loved ones and capture precious moments during and after the birth.

2. **Supportive Items:** Consider any additional items that would provide support and comfort for both you and your partner during labor and after birth. This could include massage oils, essential oils for relaxation, a soothing playlist, or any other items that help create a calming atmosphere.

The hospital bag is a physical representation of your preparedness and anticipation for your baby's arrival. By ensuring that it contains all the essentials, you are setting yourselves up for a smoother and more comfortable hospital experience. Keep the bag easily accessible in the weeks leading up to the due date, and don't forget to include any specific items or preferences your partner may have for her comfort during labor and recovery.

Chapter 6:

Labor and Delivery

The moment you've been eagerly anticipating has arrived – the day your baby will make their grand entrance into the world. The pinnacle of months of planning, joy, and, yes, a little bit of worry, is labor and delivery. As an expectant father, your role during this extraordinary journey is pivotal

Supporting Your Partner

Before the actual process of labor begins, it's essential to emphasize the critical role of support that you, as an expectant father, will play. You are not merely an observer; you are an active participant, a pillar of strength, and the calming presence that your partner needs during this intense and transformative experience.

Emotional Support

Labor can be an emotionally intense journey. Your partner might undergo a range of emotions, spanning from excitement and eager anticipation to anxiety and fear. Your primary role is to be a calming and reassuring presence. Encourage her, listen to her, and let her know that you are always available to her. Your consistent emotional support can have a profound effect on her capacity to navigate the difficulties of labor.

Advocate

In the midst of the chaos of a hospital or birthing center, your partner might not always be able to advocate for her preferences and needs. Your role includes ensuring that her birth plan and wishes are respected and communicated to the healthcare team. Be her voice when she might not be able to express her desires clearly, ensuring that her choices are acknowledged and honored.

Physical Comfort

During labor, offering physical comfort measures can provide immense relief. Simple gestures like massages, counterpressure on her back, and suggesting different positions can help alleviate pain and tension. Providing water, snacks, and cool washcloths can also contribute to her comfort. Your direct assistance can have a big impact on her experience in general.

Stay Informed

Understanding the progress of labor and any medical interventions is vital. Make sure you understand the decisions being made during the labor process by asking questions, getting explanation, and asking questions. Being informed allows you to actively participate in the decision-making process, ensuring that both you and your partner are comfortable with the choices being made.

The Big Day Arrives

The arrival of the big day, the day you've been eagerly anticipating, can be unpredictable. Labor can commence suddenly or gradually, and its onset varies from person to person. Here's what you need to know about the moments leading up to labor:

Recognizing the Signs of Labor

The onset of labor is a unique and unpredictable experience for each expectant mother. Knowing the telltale indications of labor is crucial if you want to be able to react quickly and give the required attention and support. Here are some common signs to watch for:

- **Contractions:** Contractions are one of the most unmistakable signs of labor. Unlike Braxton Hicks contractions, which are often irregular and painless, true labor contractions are regular, increasingly frequent, and more intense. They may begin as mild discomfort and gradually become stronger and more regular.

- **Water Breaking:** When your partner's water breaks, that's another telltale symptom of labor. This is the rupture of the amniotic sac, which releases amniotic fluid. The fluid is usually clear and odorless. If your partner experiences this, it's a definite indication that labor has begun.
- **Bloody Show:** A "bloody show" refers to the passage of a small amount of blood-tinged mucus from the cervix. It can be a precursor to labor and indicates that the cervix is beginning to change and dilate.
- **Backache and Pelvic Pressure:** Some women experience lower back pain and increased pelvic pressure as labor approaches. These sensations can be a result of the baby's position and the pressure on the cervix.
- **Change in Cervical Dilation and Effacement:** Your healthcare provider may have been monitoring your partner's cervical dilation and effacement during prenatal checkups. A noticeable change or progression in these measurements can indicate that labor is imminent.

Timing Contractions

Once you notice the onset of contractions, it's crucial to begin timing them. Timing contractions allows you to track their frequency, duration, and regularity, providing valuable information about the progress of labor. Here's how to time contractions effectively:

1. **Start the Timer:** Use a stopwatch, smartphone app, or a simple clock with a second hand to measure the duration of each contraction. Prepare a notepad or notebook to write down the times.

2. **Note the Beginning and End:** Start keeping track of the time between one contraction and the next. Record the time when a contraction begins and when it ends. This will provide you with the contraction's duration.

3. **Measure Frequency:** After timing a few contractions, observe how often they occur. Keep track of the interval between one contraction's beginning and the next.. This will give you the frequency.

4. **Regular Contractions:** Actual labor contractions are growing mor. In the early stages, they may be around 20 to 30 minutes apart, but they will become more frequent as labor progresses.

5. **Increasing Intensity:** The intensity and frequency of contractions increase as labor progresses. The interval between contractions typically shortens to around 5 minutes or less in active labor.

Contacting the Healthcare Provider

Knowing when to call your healthcare provider, go to the hospital, or go to a birthing center depends on how well you can timing your contractions. The guidelines for when to make the call may depend based on your healthcare provider's recommendations and the specific details of your pregnancy. However, here are some general considerations:

- **Contractions**: If your partner is experiencing regular contractions that last around 60 seconds and occur at 5-minute intervals (or as advised by your healthcare provider), it's typically time to contact the healthcare provider or go to the hospital.
- **Water Breaking**: If your partner's water breaks, contact the healthcare provider immediately, even if she isn't experiencing contractions yet. They will offer direction for the following actions.
- **Bloody Show**: If your partner experiences a significant bloody show or observes changes in cervical dilation and effacement during a routine prenatal checkup, it is recommended that the patient get in touch with their healthcare physician to address the current predicament.
- **Decreased Fetal Movement**: If your partner notices a significant decrease in fetal movement or any other concerns related to the baby's well-being, contact the healthcare provider for guidance.

Maintaining communication with your healthcare provider is crucial throughout the labor process. They can offer invaluable guidance and ensure you receive the necessary care and support.

What to Expect During Labor

Labor is divided into three main stages, each with its own distinct characteristics. Understanding these stages will help you navigate the journey more confidently:

1. First Stage: Early Labor and Active Labor

Early Labor: Early labor is the initial phase of contractions. Contractions are usually mild and irregular, and your partner may still be able to engage in activities and speak during contractions. This stage can last for several hours, and it's a crucial time for your partner to conserve energy and stay hydrated.

Active Labor: This stage of labor is characterized by the onset of more frequent and powerful contractions. Contractions become regular, lasting around 45 to 60 seconds with a 5-minute interval between them. This stage can last for several hours as well. Your partner will require increased support and focus during this phase, as the intensity of contractions escalates.

2. Second Stage: Transition and Pushing

Transition: The transition phase is often regarded as the most challenging part of labor. Intense and frequent contractions occur every two to five minutes. It's common for women to feel overwhelmed during this stage, both physically and emotionally. Your calming presence and encouragement are essential in helping your partner cope with the intensity of contractions.

Pushing: The second stage culminates in the urge to push. In order to force the baby down the birth canal, your partner will cooperate with the contractions. This stage varies in duration but is typically shorter than the previous stages. Your role here is to provide unwavering support, assist with breathing techniques, and offer encouragement. Your presence gives her the strength to endure the physical demands of pushing.

3. Third Stage: Birth of the Placenta

After the Baby is Born: The placenta, a critical organ that provided nourishment to the infant throughout pregnancy, is delivered over the third stage of labor and delivery. Contractions continue after the baby is born, helping the placenta detach from the uterine wall. Your partner may experience additional contractions, albeit milder, during this stage. The healthcare team will monitor her closely to ensure that the placenta is delivered entirely, signifying the completion of the birthing process.

Providing Emotional Support

Emotional support during labor and delivery is of paramount importance. The intensity of the experience, coupled with the anticipation of meeting the baby, can evoke a wide range of emotions. Your role as a source of emotional comfort is invaluable. Here are ways you can provide the emotional support your partner needs:

1. **Stay Calm and Reassuring**: Maintain a calm and reassuring presence, even if you are feeling anxious or nervous. Your partner will draw strength from your composure. Your steady demeanor can provide a sense of stability amidst the intensity of labor.

2. **Encouragement: Express** words of support and gratitude. Remind your partner that she is strong, resilient, and capable. Acknowledge her efforts and express your confidence in her ability to navigate the challenges of labor. Your positive words can boost her morale and instill confidence.

3. **Use Affirmations:** If you and your partner have practiced affirmations during pregnancy, this is the perfect time to use them. Calm and concentration can be achieved with the aid of positive affirmations. Repeat affirmations together,

reinforcing the belief in her body's ability to give birth. Affirmations serve as powerful mental tools during labor.

4. **Practice Active Listening:** As you pay close attention to your lover. She may need to communicate her emotions, worries, and fears during labor. As you listen to her with patience and empathy, let her express her feelings without passing judgment. Confirm her experiences and provide comfort.

5. **Provide Distraction:** Distraction can be a useful coping mechanism during labor, particularly during the early stages. Engage in conversation, play soothing music, or provide a focal point for your partner to concentrate on during contractions. Gentle distractions can help her relax between contractions and provide moments of respite.

6. **Keep Your Sense of Humor:** A well-timed joke or a lighthearted comment can assist reduce stress and foster a calm environment. Laughter has a remarkable ability to reduce stress and release endorphins, which can be particularly beneficial during labor's more challenging moments.

The First Moments with Your Baby

The moment your baby is born is an awe-inspiring and life-changing experience, unlike any other. It's a moment filled with profound emotions, from overwhelming joy and relief to deep wonder and a sense of awe. As an expectant father, your role during these first moments is to be present, supportive, and ready to embrace your newborn.

Cutting the Umbilical Cord

One of the significant moments that often falls to the expectant father is the opportunity to cut the baby's umbilical cord. This gesture is indicative of the baby's departure from the womb and their beginning of an independent life. Here's what you need to know about cutting the umbilical cord:

- **Discuss Your Preference:** Before the birth, discuss your preference regarding cutting the cord with your partner and the healthcare provider. Some fathers choose to cut the cord, while others may prefer not to. It's imperative that you express your desires beforehand.
- **Timing:** The exact circumstances surrounding the birth determine when to cut the cord. In certain instances, the medical professional might decide to hold off on clamping and cutting the cord for a few minutes in order to facilitate delayed cord clamping, which may enhance the baby's health. You will be guided through the procedure by your healthcare provider..
- **Sterile Environment:** Cutting the cord is typically done in a sterile environment, ensuring the baby's safety. The healthcare provider will provide you with sterilized scissors or clamps for the procedure.
- **Symbolic Act:** Cutting the cord is a symbolic gesture that signifies your active involvement in the birth process and your commitment to your newborn. It is a time of bonding and crossing over from the womb to the outside world.

Skin-to-Skin Contact

Promoting immediate skin-to-skin contact with your baby is highly recommended and offers numerous benefits for both the baby and the parents. This method allows for close contact by placing the infant right on the naked chest of the mother or father. Here's why skin-to-skin contact is so significant:

- **Bonding:** Skin-to-skin contact promotes bonding between the baby and the parent. It gives the infant a sense of security and an instant bond.
- **Temperature Regulation:** Newborns are particularly sensitive to temperature changes. Skin-to-skin contact helps control the baby's body temp., ensuring they stay warm and comfortable.
- **Stabilizing Vital Signs:** Skin-to-skin contact can help stabilize the baby's vital signs, including heart rate and breathing rate. It provides a soothing and calming effect.

- **Initiating Breastfeeding:** Skin-to-skin contact is often a precursor to breastfeeding. The infant may instinctively seek out the breast and start nursing as soon as they are placed on the mother's chest.
- **Comfort and Security:** Babies feel safe and secure when held skin-to-skin. It offers consolation and security as the baby leaves the womb and enters the outside world.

If your partner is unable to hold the baby immediately after birth, you can take on this role. Skin-to-skin contact is a beautiful way for fathers to connect with their newborns and create lasting bonds.

Support for Breastfeeding

If your partner plans to breastfeed, your support during the baby's first feeding is invaluable. Assist with latching and positioning as needed. Encourage and reassure her as she begins this essential bonding experience with your newborn. Your involvement can make the breastfeeding journey smoother and more enjoyable.

Bonding and Connection

The first moments with your newborn are a time of profound connection and bonding. Here are some ways to foster this special bond:

- **Gentle Touch:** Gently cradle and hold your baby. Make eye contact, stroke their tiny hands and feet, and offer soothing words. These gentle gestures create a sense of security and comfort.
- **Speak to Your Baby:** Talk to your baby in a soothing and comforting tone. Infants react to the sound of their parents' voices, thus it can be comforting for them to hear you speak.
- **Remain Present**: Give your infant your whole attention. Remain Present: Give your infant your whole attention. Set aside gadgets like cellphones and other distractions so you can concentrate on these priceless moments of intimacy.
- **Skin-to-Skin Contact:** Continue to engage in skin-to-skin contact whenever possible. There's no feeling of comfort and intimacy like it does.

- **Share in the Joy:** Share in the joy and wonder of welcoming your baby into the world with your partner. Express your love and gratitude for this incredible moment and the beautiful journey of parenthood that lies ahead.

Remember to cherish these first moments, for they are the beginning of a beautiful journey into the world of parenthood.

Chapter 7:

The Postpartum Period

Often referred to as the "fourth trimester," the postpartum period is an important time in your journey as a new parent. This is a time of adjustment, transformation, and bonding as you adapt to the new dynamics of your family with the arrival of your newborn.

Becoming a Parent

The journey into parenthood is a profound and transformative experience that reshapes every facet of your life. From the moment you learn of the impending arrival of your little one, your identity, priorities, and responsibilities undergo a significant shift. As you prepare to embrace the role of a parent, it's essential to navigate this transformation with self-awareness, open communication with your partner, and a commitment to nurturing the bonds that will shape your family's future.

Self-Reflection and Communication

Becoming a parent often prompts a period of self-reflection. You begin to contemplate your values, beliefs, and expectations regarding parenthood. This introspection is a crucial step as it helps you better understand your own desires and goals in raising a child. Examine your thoughts, feelings, and goals for a while. You can gain important understanding of your parenting style by thinking back on your own upbringing and experiences with your parents.

Keeping lines of communication open and honest with your partner is equally crucial. Share your thoughts, hopes, and concerns about parenthood. These discussions can highlight areas of agreement as well as those where you might need to make concessions or find solutions. As you travel together, it's critical that you have the same understanding.

Clarifying Roles and Responsibilities

As you prepare for your baby's arrival, it's crucial to clarify the roles and responsibilities each parent will assume. This includes everything from caregiving tasks like diaper changes, feedings, and bedtime routines to household chores and financial planning. Ensuring that both couples actively participate in the child's care and upbringing is ensured by setting clear expectations.

Additionally, it is crucial to realize that the roles may change as the child develops. Flexibility and adaptability in your parenting roles will help you navigate the changing demands of parenthood successfully. Maintaining open lines of communication with your spouse is essential to making sure that you both feel appreciated and supported in your roles as parents.

Paternal Bonding

Building a strong bond with your child is one of the most rewarding aspects of parenthood. The connection you establish in the early days and months can have a lasting impact on your child's sense of security and attachment. You are an important part of this process as an expectant father.

Invest time in bonding activities and quality time with your newborn. Skin-to-skin contact is a powerful way to establish a connection and provide comfort. Take an active role in providing your child with care, including feeding, changing diapers, and comforting them. These interactions foster trust and emotional closeness.

Remember that bonding is an ongoing journey that extends beyond infancy. As your child grows, your involvement, presence, and guidance will continue to shape the parent-child relationship. Embrace this role with love, patience, and a commitment to being a supportive and nurturing parent.

Parenting Support

Parenting is a journey filled with both joys and challenges. Seeking support and guidance from experienced parents, friends, or parenting classes can be immensely valuable. Gaining insight from the experiences and knowledge of others can make navigating the particular intricacies of parenthood easier for you.

Think about participating in online communities or parenting groups where you may exchange experiences and gain knowledge from others. Parenthood is a shared journey, and the collective wisdom of the parenting community can provide valuable insights and reassurance during times of uncertainty.

Self-Care

In the midst of caring for your child, it's easy to neglect self-care. Putting your physical and emotional health first, though, is necessary if you want to be the greatest parent possible. Make sure you schedule time for rest, exercise, and mental and physical rejuvenation.

Self-care is an essential behavior, not a selfish one. A parent who is emotionally stable and gets enough sleep is better able to provide their child the love, care, and support they need. Embrace this aspect of your role as a parent with the understanding that caring for yourself is an act of love for your family as well.

The Arrival of Your Newborn

The arrival of your newborn brings joy and excitement, along with a shift in your daily routine. Adjusting to this new routine can be challenging, but with time and patience, you will find a rhythm that works for your family. Here's what to expect:

Feeding Schedule

Newborns have demanding feeding schedules, typically needing to feed every 2-3 hours. This is something that you and your spouse need to plan and share, whether you are nursing or using a bottle. This allows both of you to get adequate rest and support each other.

Sleep Patterns

Newborns may only sleep for brief amounts of time during the day or night due to their erratic sleep patterns. Be prepared for sleep deprivation, and consider taking short naps when your baby sleeps to help you catch up on rest. Understanding that this phase is temporary can provide some relief.

Diaper Changes

Frequent diaper changes are a part of caring for a newborn. This task offers an opportunity for bonding and caregiving. Make sure that everything you need is close at hand, such as wipes, diapers, and a secure place to change.

Comfort and Soothing

Babies often require comfort and soothing, especially when they are fussy. Gentle rocking, swaddling, and using a pacifier can help calm a fussy baby. Since each baby's cues are unique, exercise patience and pay attention to them.

Monitoring Health

Regular check-ups with the pediatrician are essential during the early weeks of your baby's life. Monitoring your baby's growth, feeding patterns, and overall health is a crucial aspect of newborn care. Keep a record of your baby's milestones and health-related information for reference.

Share Responsibilities

Encourage shared responsibilities with your partner. While one parent may take the lead in certain caregiving tasks, such as breastfeeding, both parents can contribute to diaper changes, burping, and soothing the baby. Effective teamwork and support are key during this period of adjustment.

Coping with Sleep Deprivation

Sleep deprivation is one of the most challenging aspects of parenthood, especially during the early months when your baby's sleep patterns are unpredictable. Being sleep deprived can make you feel drained emotionally, agitated, and tired. However, with patience, understanding, and the right strategies, you can cope effectively with sleep deprivation and support each other as parents.

Understanding Newborn Sleep Patterns

Newborns have undeveloped circadian rhythms, meaning they don't distinguish between day and night. They sleep in short cycles, typically ranging from two to four hours. As a result, new parents often find themselves waking multiple times during the night to feed, change diapers, or soothe their baby.

Shift Sleeping

One effective strategy to cope with sleep deprivation is to establish a shift sleeping routine with your partner. Both parents can receive longer stretches of uninterrupted sleep if they alternate nighttime baby care. For example, one parent can handle the early evening and the other the late-night feedings, allowing each parent to have a few hours of continuous sleep.

Napping and Resting During the Day

While your baby naps during the day, make it a priority to rest as well. Even short naps can help alleviate some of the sleep debt. If possible, synchronize your naps so that you both get a chance to rest during the day. Creating a calm and soothing environment can aid relaxation, making it easier to nap during the day.

Accepting Help

Do not be reluctant to accept assistance from close friends and relatives. If someone offers to look after the child for a few hours, use the time to relax. It's natural to want to do everything yourself, but accepting help is not a sign of weakness—it's a practical way to ensure you get the rest you need. Whether it's a friend preparing a meal or a family member taking care of the baby, these gestures of support can make a significant difference.

Create a Sleep-Conducive Environment

For your baby, creating a sleep-conducive environment is essential for improving nighttime sleep patterns. Create a pattern for your baby's bedtime that will serve as a cue to him or her that it is time to sleep. This may comprise dimming the lights, soothing activities like reading or gentle rocking, and maintaining a consistent bedtime.

For yourself, it's equally important to create a sleep-friendly environment. Make sure the area where you sleep is cozy, quiet, and dark. You may want to contemplate the use of blackout curtains and white noise machines to establish an environment that fosters restful sleep.

Limit Screen Time

You could find it harder to fall asleep because of the blue light that is emitted from computer screens. Reduce the amount of time spent in front of electronic screens prior to going to bed, particularly in the hour prior to going to bed. Rather, try engaging in relaxing activities like reading a book, having a warm bath, or exercising relaxation strategies like deep breathing. These are going to put you at rest.

Prioritizing Self-Care

Making Self-Care a Priority It's simple to put your personal health last when tending to your newborn. However, self-care is essential for managing sleep deprivation. Take part in stress-relieving and relaxing activities. Whether it's taking a leisurely walk, practicing mindfulness meditation, or enjoying a hobby, make time for activities that bring you joy and calmness.

Communicating Openly

Speaking Honestly Keep lines of communication open regarding your feelings with your companion. Share your emotions, frustrations, and challenges related to sleep deprivation. By expressing your concerns, you create a supportive environment where both partners can empathize and work together to find solutions.

Seeking Professional Support

If your lack of sleep gets overpowering and starts to seriously damage your ability to function normally throughout the day, you should think about getting some professional assistance. You may benefit from the direction of a therapist, counselor, or support group in addition to having a secure environment in which to communicate your emotions. Talking to a trained professional or individuals who have been through something similar to what you're going through can often offer helpful insights and ideas for overcoming obstacles.

Bonding with Your Baby

Building a strong bond with your baby is an essential aspect of parenthood. The bond you create in these early months sets the foundation for a loving and secure relationship. Here are ways to strengthen your connection:

Skin-to-Skin Contact

After the first few days after giving birth, keep your infant close to your skin. This practice fosters attachment and provides comfort. It's not limited to the newborn phase and can be continued as your baby grows.

Eye Contact and Interaction

Maintain eye contact and participate in engaging activities with your infant. Play games like nursery rhymes or peek-a-boo. Your baby's responses, even in the form of coos and smiles, are signs of connection and recognition.

Cuddling and Holding

Hold and cuddle your baby frequently. Babies thrive on physical closeness and the feeling of being held securely. These moments of physical affection provide comfort and reassurance.

Talking and Singing

Talk to your child all day long. Describe what you are doing, share stories, or simply have conversations. Babies are attentive to the sound of their parents' voices, and hearing your voice can be reassuring. You and your child can both find it relaxing and joyful to sing lullabies or songs.

Respond to Cue

Observe your baby's wants and cues carefully. Respond promptly to hunger, discomfort, or the need for comfort. This responsiveness builds trust and security, reinforcing your role as a source of safety and care.

Baby-Wearing

To keep your baby close while you go about your everyday business, think considering utilizing a baby carrier or sling. Baby-wearing promotes bonding and allows your baby to be part of your routines, whether you're going for a walk or doing household tasks.

Enjoy Everyday Moments

Cherish everyday moments with your baby. These can be as simple as bath time, feeding, or cuddling before bedtime. These moments of connection are precious and contribute to your baby's sense of being loved and cherished.

Maintaining Intimacy

Parenthood is a journey that profoundly transforms your life and reshapes your priorities. It is imperative that you keep in mind that maintaining your relationship with your spouse is just as important as taking this thrilling journey. Maintaining intimacy, both emotional and physical, contributes to a healthy and fulfilling partnership as you navigate the challenges and joys of parenthood together.

Communication is Key

The arrival of a newborn brings changes to your daily routines, sleep patterns, and responsibilities. It's critical to discuss your needs, desires, and experiences with your spouse in an honest and open manner.

Share your thoughts, concerns, and aspirations regarding parenthood. Discuss how these changes are affecting you personally and as a couple. Regular check-ins can help you both stay attuned to each other's emotions and provide support when needed. Recall that effective communication requires both empathy and attentive listening.

Quality Time Together

The demands of caring for a newborn can make it challenging to find time for each other, but quality over quantity is key. Make an attempt to spend quality time with your partner, even if it's only for a short while. Plan date nights, enjoy a quiet dinner at home, or simply engage in conversations that deepen your connection.

In the early stages of parenthood, you might have to find inventive ways to spend your time with your child. Include your baby in your activities when possible, such as taking a walk with the stroller or having a picnic in the park. Prioritizing one another in the midst of everyday obligations is crucial.

Support and Acknowledgment

Supporting each other's roles and efforts as parents is a fundamental aspect of maintaining intimacy. No matter how tiny, recognize and value your partner's contributions. Express gratitude for the support and care you provide for each other and your child.

Recognize that parenthood often involves moments of doubt and insecurity. Be each other's cheerleader, offering encouragement and reassurance. Your unwavering support can boost your partner's confidence and strengthen your emotional bond.

Respect Each Other's Needs

It's normal for both you and your partner to have individual needs and priorities during this phase. Parenthood can bring about physical and emotional changes, and your responses to these changes may differ. Respect each other's needs and boundaries.

Understanding that your physical intimacy may change temporarily after the birth of your child is essential. Your partner's body may need time to heal, and her energy levels might fluctuate. Approach the topic of physical intimacy with sensitivity and empathy, discussing your desires and concerns openly.

Seek Professional Help if Needed

If you discover that the difficulties of motherhood are severely affecting your relationship, don't be afraid to get expert assistance. Couples counseling or therapy may offer helpful direction and support for the relationship. The emotional demands of parenting can be difficult to manage, but getting help from a therapist can be of great assistance in this endeavor, resolving any lingering issues, and formulating strategies to sustain intimacy.

Recall that preserving closeness is a continuous process that calls for tolerance, understanding, and flexibility. The love and connection you share with your partner are essential not only for your relationship but also for providing a stable and nurturing environment for your child.

Chapter 8:

Future Dad's Toolkit

Becoming a father is a momentous event, filled with both excitement and challenges. As you prepare to welcome your little one into the world, equipping yourself with practical knowledge and resources is essential. The Future Dad's Toolkit is your comprehensive guide, offering practical advice, insights into essential baby gear, tips on managing parental leave and work-life balance, budgeting for parenthood, and guidance on preparing emotionally for the transformative journey ahead.

Practical Advice

It takes a combination of patience, adaptability, and preparation to handle the challenges of parenthood. Here are some practical pieces of advice to help you thrive in your new role as a dad:

1. **Educate Yourself:** Read books, attend parenting classes, and engage with online resources. Understanding the stages of your baby's development, basic caregiving skills, and parenting techniques can boost your confidence and readiness.

2. **Be Hands-On:** Actively participate in caregiving tasks, from diaper changes to feeding sessions. Your engagement improves the relationship you have with your child and gives your partner important support.

3. **Practice Patience:** Parenthood is a learning curve for both you and your baby. Have patience with your partner, your child, and yourself. Making errors and growing from them is normal.

4. **Support Your Partner:** Pregnancy, childbirth, and the postpartum recovery period can pose physical and emotional challenges for your partner. Provide her with emotional support, a helpful hand, and attentive listening to her worries and feelings.

5. **Prioritize Self-Care:** Parental responsibilities can be overwhelming. Remember to take breaks, engage in activities you enjoy, and maintain your social connections. Taking care of your own well-being equips you to be a better parent.

Essential Baby Gear

Equipping your home with the necessary baby gear guarantees a safe and cozy environment for your newborn. Here's a rundown of the must-have items:

- **Crib or Bassinet:** Provide a secure sleeping space for your baby. Verify that the crib satisfies safety requirements and is devoid of any toys or soft bedding.
- **Diapers and Changing Supplies:** Stock up on diaper rash cream, diapers, wipes, and a changing pad. Create a designated changing station for convenience.
- **Clothing:** Purchase soft, comfortable onesies, sleepers, socks, and hats. Newborns grow quickly, so have a variety of sizes on hand.
- **Feeding Supplies:** Whether breastfeeding or formula-feeding, invest in nursing bras, breast pads, bottles, nipples, formula (if needed), and a breast pump for expressing milk.
- **Car Seat:** One non-negotiable safety requirement is a well mounted car seat. Research and choose a car seat that fits your vehicle and meets safety standards.
- **Stroller:** Whether you want a sturdy jogging stroller or a lightweight, portable stroller, choose the one that best fits your needs.
- **Baby Carrier:** Baby carriers promote bonding and allow for hands-free mobility. Select a carrier that will adequately support your baby's growing spine.
- **Baby Monitor:** You can monitor your kid from another room with peace of mind if you have a baby monitor with audio and video capabilities.

- **Health and Safety Items:** Include a thermometer, baby nail clippers, a nasal aspirator, baby-friendly laundry detergent, and a first-aid kit in your baby gear arsenal.

Parental Leave and Work-Life Balance

Balancing the responsibilities of parenthood with a demanding career can be one of the most challenging aspects of becoming a father. Parental leave policies and achieving a sustainable work-life balance are crucial factors that significantly impact your ability to support your family while nurturing your relationship with your partner and child.

Understanding Parental Leave Policies

Understanding your rights and entitlements regarding parental leave is essential. Familiarize yourself with the parental leave policies in your country and workplace. Paternity leave is a benefit that several nations provide, enabling fathers to take time out of work to care for their newborns. Be aware of the duration of the leave, whether it is paid or unpaid, and the process for requesting leave.

In some regions, parental leave policies have evolved to be more inclusive, recognizing the importance of fathers in caregiving roles. Some countries provide shared parental leave options, allowing both parents to divide the leave period according to their needs and preferences.

Planning Your Parental Leave

Planning your parental leave involves thoughtful consideration of your partner's needs, your baby's well-being, and your own mental and physical health. Here are some strategies to consider:

- **Communication with Your Employer:** Initiate open communication with your employer about your intention to take parental leave. Provide ample notice, discuss the duration of your leave, and explore any flexible work arrangements that can ease the transition.

- **Coordinate with Your Partner:** Collaborate with your partner to plan your leave periods strategically. Coordinate your schedules to ensure continuous care for your baby. This cooperative strategy enables both parents to successfully manage their roles as caregivers and workers.
- **Utilize Family and Support Networks:** Lean on your family and support networks during your parental leave. Having assistance from relatives or close friends can provide relief and allow you and your partner to take breaks and rest.

Achieving Work-Life Balance:

It is crucial for both your general health and your capacity to be there for your family that you find a way to strike a healthy balance between your job life and your personal life. Here are some tips to strike a balance between your career and family life:

- **Set Boundaries:** Clearly define your work hours and adhere to them as much as possible. Steer clear of overworking, as this can cause burnout and hinder your ability to spend quality time with your family.
- **Prioritize Tasks:** Prioritize your tasks at work and home. Focus on completing high-priority tasks efficiently. As much as possible, assign chores to others for both your household and your place of employment.
- **Embrace Flexible Work Arrangements:** Examine the flexible work options that your company has, such as remote work, adjustable hours, or shortened workweeks. These arrangements can allow you the freedom you need to successfully manage your personal and professional lives.
- **Practice Self-Care:** If you want to maintain the best possible mental and physical health, you should put yourself first. Maintain a regular exercise routine, ensure you are getting enough rest, and make time for the things that offer you joy and relaxation. Taking care of oneself makes it easier for you to manage the responsibilities of both parenthood and the workplace.
- **Spending Quality Time with Family:** Be attentive and involved when spending time with your family.. Building strong ties and making treasured experiences with

your child and partner requires spending quality time together. Limit distractions during family time to fully enjoy the moments together.

- **Frequent Check-Ins:** Evaluate the harmony between work and family life by checking in with your spouse on a frequent basis. Talk about any difficulties or changes that must be made to make sure that each partner feels encouraged and appreciated in their jobs.

Navigating parental leave and work-life balance as a father requires careful planning, communication, and flexibility. Remember that your presence and support in your child's life are invaluable, and finding the right balance is a worthy pursuit for the well-being of your family.

Budgeting for Parenthood

Parenthood brings new financial responsibilities. Thoughtful budgeting and financial planning can provide stability and security for your growing family:

1. **Create a Baby Budget:** Assess your current financial situation and create a budget specifically tailored to the needs of your expanding family. Account for medical expenses, baby gear, childcare, and ongoing baby-related costs.

2. **Emergency Fund:** Increase or expand your emergency savings. Maintaining a financial safety net offers peace of mind and protects your family from unforeseen financial burdens.

3. **Health Insurance:** Review your health insurance coverage. Understand the costs related to childbirth, well-baby check-ups, vaccinations, and pediatric care. Ensure your insurance plan adequately covers these expenses.

4. **Childcare Costs:** Research childcare options and associated costs. Set aside money for this important investment whether you decide on family care, daycare, or a nanny.

5. **Review and Modify**: Continually assess your financial objectives and budget. Parenthood may necessitate adjustments in your spending habits and savings priorities. Be proactive in adapting your financial plan to meet your family's needs.

Preparing for Parenthood

As you get ready for the birth of your child, there are a few important things that you as an expectant father need to think about.

Educating Yourself

One of the most valuable resources on your journey to parenthood is knowledge. Spend some time learning about delivery, pregnancy, and infant care. Attend prenatal classes with your partner, where you can learn about the stages of pregnancy, labor and delivery processes, and newborn care techniques. Books, online resources, and discussions with experienced parents can provide additional insights.

Understanding the changes your partner's body will undergo during pregnancy and the challenges she might face can enhance your empathy and support. Being knowledgeable about childbirth options and medical interventions can empower you to be an active and informed advocate for your partner's preferences during labor and delivery.

Emotional Preparation

Parenthood is not just about the physical care of a child; it's also about emotional readiness and building a strong foundation for your family. Initiate candid and sincere dialogues with your partner about your expectations, concerns, and hopes concerning parenthood. Discuss your parenting styles, beliefs, and values, and find common ground.

Prepare emotionally for the changes parenthood will bring to your relationship with your partner. Discuss how you will navigate challenges together, maintain intimacy, and support each other emotionally. Be prepared for the shifts in your daily routines, sleep patterns, and personal time. Adaptability and flexibility are crucial traits to have when accepting the unpredictability of parenting.

Chapter 9:

Your New Identity

Embracing Fatherhood

Being a father is a special and incredibly intimate experience. It's a process of providing for, advising, and encouraging your child as they mature. It's about being there to celebrate their triumphs and console them during their setbacks. It's a role filled with responsibilities and challenges, but it's also one that brings immeasurable joy and fulfillment.

As a father, you play a vital role in your child's life. Your presence, love, and guidance shape their sense of security and self-esteem. Your role goes beyond providing for their physical needs; it's about being a source of emotional support, a mentor, and a role model.

The transition into fatherhood may not always be smooth, and it can come with a range of emotions. You may feel excitement, anxiety, uncertainty, and profound love, often all at once. Embracing fatherhood means accepting these emotions and understanding that it's a journey filled with growth and learning.

Shifting Priorities

Parenthood inevitably brings a shift in priorities. Your child's needs and well-being become your foremost concern. Your new normal consists of diaper changes, late-night feedings, and soothing cries. These adjustments might be difficult, but they are also incredibly fulfilling.

Accepting this change means realizing that it's a normal phase of being a parent. Prioritizing your child's needs doesn't mean neglecting your own Instead, the key is to strike a balance that lets you take care of your child and yourself. Finding this balance is not always simple, and you might need to make adjustments as you go. But keep in mind that caring for yourself is not selfish; rather, it's essential for your own health and your capacity to be a loving and supporting parent. Reconnecting with Your Partner

As your focus shifts to your child, it's essential not to neglect your relationship with your partner. Parenthood can be all-consuming, but maintaining a strong and loving partnership is vital for the well-being of your family.

The early months of parenthood can be particularly challenging for couples as they navigate the sleepless nights and the demands of caring for a newborn. It's critical to discuss your needs and feelings with your partner in an honest and open manner. Share your experiences, your joys, and your frustrations. You and your partner can weather the storms of early motherhood together if you maintain open channels of communication.

In addition to communication, schedule regular date nights or moments of connection with your partner. Even simple gestures like a heartfelt conversation, holding hands, or sharing a laugh can strengthen your bond. Keep in mind that your connection is the cornerstone of your family and that it must be nurtured.

Self-Care for New Dads

Amidst the demands of fatherhood, self-care often takes a backseat. But maintaining your physical and mental health is crucial for your own benefit as well as your capacity to be a loving and supporting parent.

1. **Prioritize Sleep:** Sleep is precious, especially in the early months of parenthood. Create a sleep schedule that allows both you and your partner to get adequate rest, even if it means taking turns caring for your baby. Insufficient sleep can affect your mood, cognitive function, and overall well-being.

2. **Healthy Lifestyle:** Maintaining a well-balanced diet and getting regular exercise are crucial for maintaining good physical health. Maintaining an active lifestyle and eating healthy might help you feel more energized and cope with stress.

3. **Seek Support:** Never be afraid to ask for help from loved ones, friends, or a therapist if you're depressed after giving birth or feeling overwhelmed. The transition to parenthood can be emotionally challenging, and it's okay to ask for help. The state of your mind has a critical role in your ability to parent successfully.

4. **Time for Hobbies:** Continue engaging in hobbies and activities you enjoy. It's essential to have moments of personal fulfillment outside of parenthood. Following your passions improves your wellbeing and provides a good example for your child by highlighting the value of self-care.

5. **Social Connections:** Maintain your social connections and friendships. Parenthood can sometimes lead to social isolation, so make an effort to stay connected with friends who provide emotional support and companionship.

6. **Mental Health:** Prioritize your mental well-being. Engage in mindfulness and stress-reduction practices to effectively manage the inevitable challenges that accompany parenthood. Meditation, deep breathing exercises, and yoga offer effective means to maintain mental equilibrium.

Building Lasting Memories

Your child's early years are full with significant events, such as when they take their first steps or say their first words. Building lasting memories involves being present for these precious moments and actively participating in your child's life.

1. **Quality Time:** Make time to spend quality time connecting with your child. Play, read, sing, and explore the world together. These interactions lay the foundation for

a strong parent-child relationship. During these times, give yourself up to distractions and be really present.

2. **Capture Moments:** Document your child's growth and development through photos and videos. You and your child will be able to cherish these memories for a long time to come.

3. **Family Traditions:** Establish family traditions and rituals that create a sense of belonging and security for your child. Whether it's a weekly family game night or a special holiday tradition, these rituals strengthen family bonds and provide a sense of continuity and stability.

4. **Create Adventures:** Embark on adventures with your child, whether it's a visit to the park, a nature hike, or a trip to the zoo. These experiences foster curiosity, creativity, and a love of exploration in your child. They also create lasting memories of shared adventures.

5. **Open Communication:** Encourage open communication with your child from an early age. Establish a space where your youngster can freely express their ideas and emotions. Have meaningful discussions, pay attention when others are speaking, and offer assistance when required.

Embracing your new identity as a father is a multifaceted journey that involves personal growth, adaptability, and a deep well of love and patience. Remember that your journey is uniquely yours, and there is no one-size-fits-all approach to fatherhood. Parenthood is an incredible adventure filled with love, laughter, and moments that will shape your child's life and your own. Embrace it with an open heart, and relish the beauty of the journey.

Chapter 10:

Common Challenges and Fears

A Troubleshooting Guide

There are many unforeseen difficulties and uncertainties in parenthood. Here's a comprehensive troubleshooting guide to help you navigate some of the common issues you might encounter:

1. **Feeding Difficulties:** If your baby is struggling with breastfeeding or bottle-feeding, seek guidance from a lactation consultant or pediatrician. They can offer direction and encouragement to make sure your child gets the nourishment they need. Remember that feeding your baby can be a bonding experience, so be patient and nurturing during this time.

2. **Sleep Issues:** Sleepless nights are a common challenge for new parents. Establish a consistent bedtime routine for your baby, create a conducive sleep environment, and take turns with your partner to handle nighttime awakenings. Additionally, think about employing age- and need-appropriate sleep-training methods with your child.

3. **Coping with Colic:** Colic can be distressing for both parents and babies. Try a variety of relaxing methods, like swaddling, soft rocking, or employing white noise generators. Arrange a consultation with your pediatrician to eliminate potential underlying medical issues, and keep in mind that colic frequently resolves on its own as your baby matures.

4. **Teething Troubles:** Babies may find teething to be painful. Provide teething toys, offer cool (not frozen) teething rings, and consider using teething gels or medications

as recommended by your pediatrician. Keep in mind that teething is a temporary phase, and your baby will eventually have a full set of teeth.

5. **Sibling Rivalry:** Handling sibling rivalry can be difficult if you have multiple children. Encourage open communication, promote fairness, and allocate individual attention to each child. To encourage a sense of participation and responsibility, think about enlisting the help of older siblings in caregiving duties.

6. **Parenting Disagreements:** It's natural for parents to have differing opinions on parenting approaches. Engage in respectful discussions with your partner to find common ground and make joint decisions about your child's upbringing. Remember that both perspectives can contribute to your child's well-rounded development.

7. **Balancing Work and Family:** It can be difficult to find the ideal work-family balance, but it's essential for your health and the happiness of your family. Communicate with your employer about flexible work options, delegate tasks at home, and form clear boundaries between work and family time. Furthermore, contemplate establishing a calendar for the family to monitor significant occasions and obligations.

Overcoming Parenting Anxiety

Parenting anxiety is a common experience for many fathers. It can be quite difficult to overcome the dread of making errors or not being a good enough parent. Here are strategies to help you overcome parenting anxiety:

1. **Educate Yourself:** Knowledge is a powerful tool. Learn about kid safety, parenting styles, and child development. Knowing what to anticipate at every turn will ease your mind and assist you in making wise choices.

2. **Seek Support:** Do not be afraid to seek support from those you know, whether it be friends, family, or support groups. Sharing your fears and concerns with others who

have been through similar experiences can provide reassurance and a sense of community.

3. **Practice Self-Compassion:** Be gentle to yourself, and realize its ok to admit that you're human and prone to error. Everyone learns as a parent, and nobody is flawless. Be as nice and sympathetic to yourself as you would be to your child if you were that child's parent. Never forget how important the love and work you put into raising your children are.

4. **Stay Mindful:** By incorporating mindfulness techniques such as meditation and deep breathing exercises, you can enhance your ability to stay in the moment and alleviate anxiety. These exercises can also help you become more emotionally resilient, which will improve your ability to handle difficult situations with composure and clarity.

5. **Communicate with Your Partner:** Share your feelings of anxiety with your partner. They might be feeling similar things, so you can help one other through difficult times. Maintaining a robust partnership during parenthood necessitates open and sincere communication.

6. **Consult Professionals:** If anxiety becomes overwhelming and begins to interfere with your daily life, consider speaking to a therapist or counselor who specializes in parenting and anxiety. They can provide tools and coping strategies tailored to your needs, helping you manage anxiety effectively.

Coping with Crying and Sleepless Nights

Crying and sleepless nights are inevitable aspects of early parenthood. Coping with these challenges requires patience, understanding, and teamwork:

1. **Understand Your Baby's Cues:** Babies communicate through cries. Learn to distinguish between your baby's different cries, which can signal hunger, tiredness, discomfort, or a need for a diaper change. Responding to their specific needs can reduce crying and help you meet their requirements more efficiently.

2. **Create a Soothing Routine:** Establish a soothing bedtime ritual for your infant to indicate that it's time to go to sleep. Turn down the lights, turn up some relaxing music, and take a warm bath or leisurely rocking. Consistency in these routines can help your baby associate them with sleep.

3. **Share Nighttime Duties:** Taking turns with your partner to handle nighttime feedings and soothing can provide each of you with much-needed rest. Support each other in managing sleepless nights, and consider expressing milk if your partner is breastfeeding to allow you to participate more actively in nighttime care.

4. **Swaddle and Use White Noise:** White noise machines can simulate the reassuring sounds of the womb, and swaddling can increase your baby's sense of security. These techniques can aid in calming your baby and promoting better sleep patterns. Be sure to follow safe swaddling practices to prevent overheating and ensure your baby's hips have room to move.

5. **Consult a Pediatrician:** See your pediatrician if your infant is sobbing excessively, continuously, or in conjunction with other worrisome signs. Ensuring you rule out any potential underlying medical concerns, such as reflux, allergies, or infections, is vital when addressing your baby's discomfort.

6. **Establish a Sleep Schedule:** As your baby gets older, work on establishing a sleep schedule that aligns with their natural sleep patterns. Consistent bedtimes and wake

times can help regulate your baby's internal clock, making sleep routines more predictable.

Juggling Career and Family Life

For many fathers, juggling the demands of job and family life is an ongoing struggle. Achieving a sense of harmony requires careful planning and communication:

1. **Set Boundaries:** Create distinct compartments for your time spent working and with family. When you're at work, focus on your responsibilities and strive to be efficient. Prioritize your family when you're at home, and try not to let work-related stress interfere with your personal life.

2. **Flexible Work Arrangements:** If your employer provides them, take advantage of flexible work arrangements like telecommuting or rearranged hours. Flexibility can help you better manage both your professional and parental duties, and it demonstrates to your employer your commitment to balancing work and family life effectively.

3. **Plan Family Time:** Schedule dedicated family time in your calendar. Whether it's family dinners, weekend outings, or bedtime routines, having set times for bonding with your child ensures that you prioritize these moments. To stay organized and monitor significant occasions and obligations, think about making a family calendar.

4. **Assign Responsibilities**: Assign your spouse the chores and childcare duties. Teamwork and open communication are vital in ensuring that both parents have time for their careers and their family. Create a list of household tasks and discuss how you can divide them fairly and efficiently.

5. **Self-Care:** If you want to maintain the best possible mental and physical health, you must put yourself first. To effectively handle stress and exhaustion, use regular

exercise, restful sleep, and relaxation techniques. Taking care of yourself ensures you have the energy and resilience to be an involved and supportive father.

6. **Seek Support:** Rely on your circle of family and friends for support when you need it. Accept offers of help and consider arranging for childcare or assistance with household tasks. Creating a solid support network can help reduce some of the stress associated with juggling work and family obligations.

7. **Embrace Adaptability:** Parenthood often comes with unexpected challenges and changes in routine. Be adaptable and resilient in responding to these shifts in your daily life. Your ability to be flexible will come in handy when juggling your parental and professional obligations.

Navigating Parenting Conflicts

Parenting conflicts can arise when you and your partner have differing opinions on how to raise your child. Effective communication and compromise are key to navigating these conflicts:

1. **Open Dialogue:** Engage in open and respectful conversations with your partner about your parenting values and goals. Understanding each other's perspectives is essential.

2. **Compromise:** Always be open to make concessions and find a happy medium. It is possible that you will need to modify the ways in which you parent in order to better match with each other's ideas.

3. **Shared Decision-Making:** Make decisions about your child's upbringing together. Whether it's discipline, educational choices, or healthcare decisions, collaborative decision-making strengthens your partnership.

4. **Seek Guidance:** If you're unable to resolve conflicts on your own, consider seeking guidance from a counselor or therapist who specializes in family dynamics and parenting. Professional support can facilitate productive discussions.

5. **Prioritize the Child's Best Interests:** Remember that your shared goal is the well-being and happiness of your child. Keeping this perspective in mind can help you navigate conflicts with a focus on what's best for your family.

Parenthood is a continuous learning experience, and with patience, support, and resilience, you can navigate these challenges and fears while creating a loving and nurturing environment for your child. Embrace the journey, knowing that you have the capacity to overcome obstacles and be the best father you can be.

Chapter 11:

The Future Dad's Support Network

As you embark on the journey of fatherhood, you're not alone in facing the challenges and joys that come with it. Building a robust support network can make all the difference in your experience as a father.

Connecting with Other Dads

Fatherhood can sometimes feel like a solitary endeavor, particularly if you're the first among your friends to embrace this new role. However, the power of camaraderie with other fathers should not be underestimated. Connecting with fellow dads can provide emotional support, a sense of belonging, and a wealth of shared experiences.

1. **Joining Parenting Groups:** Consider seeking out local parenting groups or associations within your community. These groups often organize gatherings, playdates, workshops, and events designed to foster connections among parents, including fathers. Being present at these events can be a great opportunity to connect with other fathers who are navigating parenthood.

2. **Participating in Parenting Classes:** Many communities offer parenting classes and workshops that cater specifically to expectant and new fathers. These classes not only equip you with valuable parenting skills but also provide an ideal setting to bond with other dads who share your stage of fatherhood.

3. **Exploring Dad-Focused Events:** Keep an eye out for dad-focused events in your area, such as dad-and-kid gatherings, father-child sports leagues, or "dads-only"

nights out. These events provide a unique space where fathers can forge meaningful connections while enjoying shared activities.

4. **Active Involvement in Your Child's Activities:** As your child grows, they will likely engage in various extracurricular activities and sports. Consider actively participating in these activities as a coach, volunteer, or enthusiast. In doing so, you not only bond with your child but also have the opportunity to interact with other dads who share similar interests.

5. **Initiate Conversations:** Don't underestimate the power of casual conversations. Whether it's at school events, pediatrician's waiting rooms, or local parks, reaching out and initiating conversations with fellow dads can lead to the establishment of meaningful connections. Saying "hello" can lead to enduring friendships.

Online Communities and Resources

In our digital age, the internet has become an invaluable resource for parents. Online communities and resources offer a vast repository of information, advice, and opportunities for interaction with other fathers.

1. **Dad Blogs and Podcasts:** Dad-focused blogs and podcasts have proliferated in recent years, offering a treasure trove of personal anecdotes, insights, and practical advice from fellow fathers. These platforms provide a sense of solidarity and can help you glean wisdom from those who have walked a similar path.

2. **Social Media Groups:** There are a plethora of parenting-related groups on social media sites like Facebook and Reddit. Joining these groups allows you to engage with a global community of parents, exchange ideas, and find support from others who understand the unique challenges and joys of fatherhood.

3. **Parenting Forums:** Numerous websites host parenting forums where dads can ask questions, share tips, and engage in discussions. These discussion boards offer a

venue for asking seasoned dads for advice and talking about a variety of parenting subjects.

4. **Online Parenting Classes:** For those who prefer online learning, there are many parenting classes specifically designed for fathers. These classes cover a diverse array of topics, ranging from newborn care to positive discipline, offering the flexibility to learn at your own pace.

5. **Parenting Apps:** Some parenting apps come equipped with features that connect you with other dads in your locality. These apps can be instrumental in arranging playdates, sharing parenting insights, and coordinating family activities, all while fostering a sense of community.

Seeking Professional Help

While connecting with other dads and accessing online resources can be immensely beneficial, there are instances when seeking professional help is both responsible and necessary for your well-being and that of your family.

1. **Postpartum Depression:** Postpartum Depression: It's important to understand that postpartum depression affects both men and women. If you or your partner is grappling with feelings of depression or overwhelming anxiety following the birth of your child, don't hesitate to reach out to a mental health professional. They can provide direction, encouragement, and a range of individualized therapy alternatives.

2. **Chronic Parenting Challenges:** Parenting, especially during the early years, can present persistent and complex challenges. If you find yourself grappling with ongoing parenting difficulties for which you can't seem to find effective solutions, consider seeking guidance from a parenting coach or therapist. These professionals can provide you with individualized plans and methods based on your unique situation.

3. **Relationship Issues:** Parenthood can put strain on your relationship with your partner, and conflicts may arise. If you're experiencing ongoing difficulties or conflicts within your relationship, couples counseling can be instrumental in helping both of you navigate these challenges, improve communication, and strengthen your bond as a couple.

4. **Child Development Concerns:** If you have concerns about your child's development, whether related to speech delays, behavioral issues, or developmental milestones, it's essential to consult with a pediatrician or child psychologist. Early intervention can be crucial in addressing these concerns and ensuring your child receives the necessary support and resources.

5. **Grief and Loss:** It can be extremely taxing to deal with a child's death or an emotionally taxing pregnancy. In these situations, seeking support from a grief counselor or therapist is essential for healing, processing your emotions, and finding ways to move forward.

Building Lifelong Friendships

One of the most remarkable aspects of fatherhood is its potential for forging lifelong friendships. As you engage in parenting activities and connect with other dads, you'll discover that shared experiences and challenges create a unique bond with fellow fathers.

1. **Shared Experiences:** Fatherhood is a shared journey, and the challenges and joys you encounter during this chapter of your life create a profound bond with other fathers. Many lifelong friendships are formed during late-night diaper changes, toddler tantrums, and heartwarming milestones.

2. **Supportive Network:** As your children grow and embark on their own journeys, having a supportive network of fellow fathers becomes invaluable. These friends can offer advice, lend a helping hand when needed, and celebrate your child's

achievements with you. You'll find that navigating the intricacies of parenthood is more manageable with a trusted group of fellow dads by your side.

3. **Creating Cherished Memories:** Spending time with your children and other fathers results in lasting memories that you'll treasure for years to come. Whether it's coaching your kids' sports team or organizing a camping trip, these shared experiences strengthen your friendships and create cherished moments for your families.

4. **Navigating Parenting Challenges Together:** Parenting isn't always easy, and having friends who understand the challenges can make a significant difference. Your fellow dads can provide practical solutions, empathetic listening, and a sense of camaraderie during tough times. Whether it's sharing tips for managing sleepless nights or offering guidance on handling teenage rebellion, your dad friends can be a source of wisdom and support.

5. **Support for Life's Journey:** The friendships forged through fatherhood extend beyond parenting. These friends become a steadfast source of support in all aspects of life. Your dad buddies are there to support you and celebrate your accomplishments, whether it's with work guidance or personal milestones and problems.

Connecting with other dads, whether through local groups, online communities, or seeking professional help when necessary, enhances your experience as a father. It provides reassurance, shared wisdom, and a sense of belonging that can ease the challenges and amplify the joys of parenthood. As you set forth on this remarkable journey, remember that you have a vast community of fathers who understand and are ready to support you every step of the way.

Conclusion

As you reach the conclusion of this guide, it's essential to take a moment to reflect on the incredible journey you are embarking upon: the journey of fatherhood. It's a journey filled with moments of joy, challenges, personal growth, and the profound privilege of nurturing a new life. While the road ahead may be marked by uncertainties and sleepless nights, it will also be illuminated by the radiant smile of your child, their first steps, and countless memories that will etch themselves into the tapestry of your life.

Celebrating Your Journey

Every father's journey is unique, but it's bound together by a shared sense of love, dedication, and commitment. Here are some key takeaways to carry with you on your journey into fatherhood:

1. **Embrace Every Moment:** Cherish every moment you spend with your child, from the first time you hold them in your arms to their first words and beyond. Before you realize it, your child will be venturing out into the world by themselves.

2. **Lean on Your Support Network:** Never be afraid to ask for help and advice from other dads, your partner, family, and friends. Parenthood is a team effort, and you're not alone on this adventure.

3. **Seek Growth in Challenges:** The challenges you face as a father are opportunities for growth. Whether it's sleepless nights, parenting conflicts, or the ups and downs of your child's development, each challenge presents a chance to learn and become a better parent.

4. **Celebrate Milestones:** Honor your child's accomplishments, no matter how modest. These achievements mark their growth and development, and they offer you a chance to reflect on your journey as a father.

5. **Practice Self-Care:** Recall that your health and your capacity to care for your child depend on you taking care of yourself. Make self-care a priority, look for downtime, and keep a healthy work-life balance.

6. **Stay Curious:** Approach becoming a parent with an open mind and an eagerness to learn. Your child is a special person with a distinct personality, and getting to know them will be an amazing lifelong experience.

7. **Love Unconditionally:** The love you have for your child is unconditional. It transcends the challenges and difficulties, and it's the foundation of your bond. Your love is a powerful force that will guide you through the ups and downs of parenting.

Resources and Further Reading

As a father, you are on a continuing journey where there is always more to learn and explore. To continue enriching your knowledge and finding inspiration on your path as a dad, consider exploring the following resources and reading materials:

1. **Books on Parenting:** Numerous books offer valuable insights into parenting. Classics such as Daniel J. Katz's "The Whole-Brain Child". Harvey Karp's "The Happiest Baby on the Block" or Siegel and Tina Payne Bryson. These books provide practical advice on understanding and nurturing your child.

2. **Online Parenting Communities:** Engage with online parenting communities and forums where you can ask questions, share experiences, and learn from other parents. Excellent places to start include websites such as What to Expect, BabyCenter, and the parenting subreddits on Reddit.

3. **Parenting Podcasts:** Parenting podcasts provide a convenient way to access advice and insights on the go. Popular podcasts like "The Longest Shortest Time," "Parenting: Difficult Conversations," and "The Dad Edge Podcast" cover a wide range of parenting topics.

4. **Local Parenting Groups:** Continue participating in local parenting groups and events in your community. These events provide a chance to network with other parents and obtain support and insights from the community.

5. **Parenting Workshops and Classes:** Look for parenting workshops and classes in your area. These educational opportunities cover a variety of parenting topics and provide a chance to interact with experts and fellow parents.

6. **Professional Parenting Counselors:** If you encounter specific challenges or wish to enhance your parenting skills, consider consulting with a parenting counselor or therapist. They can provide tailored guidance and strategies.

7. **Dad Blogs and Magazines:** Explore dad-focused blogs and magazines that delve into the experiences of modern fathers. Websites like "Fatherly," "The Dad Website," and "Dad 2.0" offer a wealth of articles and stories about fatherhood.

8. **Parenting Apps:** Many parenting apps offer features that can assist you in various aspects of parenthood, from tracking your child's developmental milestones to managing schedules and sleep routines.

To sum up, becoming a father is an incredible experience full of love, development, and innumerable priceless moments. Embrace this journey with an open heart and a curious mind, knowing that you have the capacity to be the loving, supportive, and nurturing father your child needs. Honor every accomplishment and difficulty because they are all intricate pieces of the lovely quilt that is parenthood. As you continue to learn, grow, and connect with other dads and parenting resources, you're not just shaping the life of your child but also creating a legacy of love and care that will endure for generations to come. Welcome to fatherhood – the most extraordinary journey of your life.

* 9 7 9 8 8 6 7 7 1 1 9 5 5 *